# An Atlas of
# Ophthalmic Trauma

# AN ATLAS OF OPHTHALMIC TRAUMA

**Thomas C Spoor** MD FACS

Professor of Ophthalmology and Neurosurgery
Kresge Eye Institute of Wayne State University
Detroit, Michigan
USA

MARTIN DUNITZ

© Martin Dunitz Ltd 1997

First published in the United Kingdom in 1997 by
Martin Dunitz Ltd
The Livery House
7–9 Pratt Street
London NW1 0AE

A CIP catalogue record for this book is available from the
British Library.

ISBN 1-85317-299-5

Composition by Scribe Design, Gillingham, Kent,
United Kingdom
Origination by Bright Arts, Hong Kong
Manufactured in Singapore by Imago

# Contents

*1*   **Introduction to ocular trauma**   1

*2*   **The ruptured globe**   21

*3*   **Anterior segment injuries: blunt ocular trauma—What happens when the eye is struck by a blunt object?**   35

*4*   **Thermal and caustic ocular trauma**   45

*5*   **Posterior segment trauma**   51
*Dean Eliott*

*6*   **Eyelid and lacrimal trauma**   67

*7*   **Neuro-ophthalmologic manifestations of cranial and ocular trauma**   95

*8*   **Penetrating orbital injuries**   115

*9*   **The inflamed orbit**   131

*10*  **Orbital fractures**   153
*Thomas C Spoor and John McHenry*

*11*  **Management of traumatic optic neuropathy**   175
*Thomas C Spoor and John McHenry*

*12*  **Appendix: Ophthalmologic emergencies**   191

     **Index**   203

# Dedication

*Deanne and Kristen — Thank you!*

# Preface

Why another book on management of ocular and adnexal trauma? Why not?

Today's residents in training are not getting the extensive experience in management of ocular, orbital and adnexal trauma that we got 10–15 years ago. Recently the chief of our trauma service was bemoaning the fact that they had not seen a ruptured globe in three months. Ten years earlier, we saw one ruptured globe a week. The ophthalmic practitioner —comprehensive ophthalmologist—rarely sees a patient with severe ocular and adnexal injuries. When one presents—what do I do? These patients are different from those walking into the ophthalmologist's office with a defined complaint. They often do not know exactly what happened to them, only that something bad has occurred, and they want it fixed. They also have no established relationship with the doctor. This makes them potential high-risk litigants if a less than excellent result is obtained.

I hope that this book, with its user-friendly, atlas format, copious illustrations, and aphorisms will provide the resident and practitioner with readily accessible information to help with the management of patients with acute ocular and adnexal injuries. This text is not intended to be the definitive word on ocular trauma. The definitive word changes as knowledge and experience increase. This atlas is intended to be a readily accessible entry point into the realm of ophthalmic trauma.

The subject matter is, of course, skewed towards oculoplastic surgery and neuro-ophthalmology. These represent my basic interests and are also understressed in many training programs. I have not gone into great detail in basic methodology of anterior segment surgery, that is, techniques for cataract removal and glaucoma filtering procedures. These techniques are basic to ophthalmic surgery and should be common knowledge even to those residents finishing 'kinder and gentler' programs, with minimal exposure to trauma.

Management of patients with acute injuries and visual loss is often perplexing, even to experienced practitioners. I hope that the information in this atlas will make management a bit easier.

# *Chapter 1* **Introduction to ocular trauma**

The physician encountering a patient with injuries in and around the eye and orbital region must ask him- or herself several key questions prior to commencing evaluation and treatment. Is the injury confined to the eye and ocular adnexa or are adjacent structures involved? Figures 1.1 and 1.2 demonstrate the relationship between the eye and the surrounding brain and sinuses. Figure 1.1 demonstrates structures adjacent to the orbit viewed in the axial plane. Medial to the orbit and separated from it by the very thin lamina papryciae is the ethmoid sinus. Following the medial orbital wall posteriorly, it becomes the medial

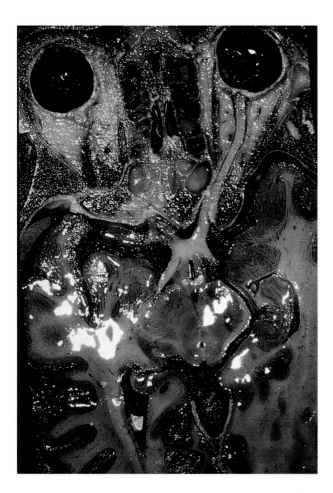

**Figure 1.1** *Axial cadaver section demonstrating adjacent orbital structures in the axial plane.*

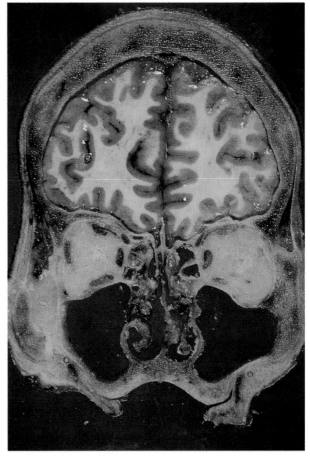

**Figure 1.2** *Coronal cadaver section demonstrating adjacent orbital structures in the coronal plane.*

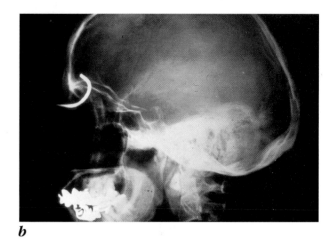

**Figure 1.3** *Metallic rod injury to the orbit completely sparing the globe but entering the adjacent anterior cranial fossa (b).*

wall of the optic canal, separating the optic nerve from the sphenoid sinus. Deep to the optic canal is the middle cranial fossa containing the optic chiasm, cavernous sinus and intracranial portion of the optic nerve. The temporal lobe of the brain lies lateral to the posterior orbit. Figure 1.2 demonstrates the relationship of the eye to the adjacent structures in the coronal plane.

Superior to the eye and orbit lies the anterior cranial fossa and the frontal sinus. Inferior lies the maxillary sinus, and medially lies the ethmoid sinus. Apparent ocular injuries might totally spare the eye, but cause significant intracranial injury (Figs 1.3(a) and (b)). Injuries to the orbital region may involve these other adjacent structures, complicating the management of these patients.

Is the brain involved? If the periocular injury has involved the eye, orbit and the brain (Fig. 1.4) management of the ocular injury must be delayed while the more significant intracranial injury is treated.

Are the sinuses involved? An injury violating the paranasal sinuses introduces a degree of contamination and may lead to infection of the eye or orbit (Fig. 1.5).

Is the eye salvageable? The eye may be completely spared in the face of very severe orbital and adnexal trauma (Fig. 1.6) or may be severely disrupted by similar trauma (Fig. 1.7). A careful, complete examination will determine the status of the eye and the

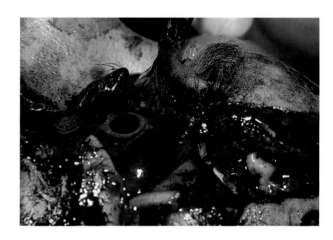

**Figure 1.4** *Periorbital injury caused by a motorboat propeller, sparing the eye but involving the eyelids and brain.*

adjacent structures. When managing patients with periorbital trauma, it is best to expect the worst, rule out significant involvement of adjacent structures, and then proceed to treat the eye.

Does this eye have visual potential, or is there no hope for any visual function? It is rather amazing the number of eyes that can be salvaged with some

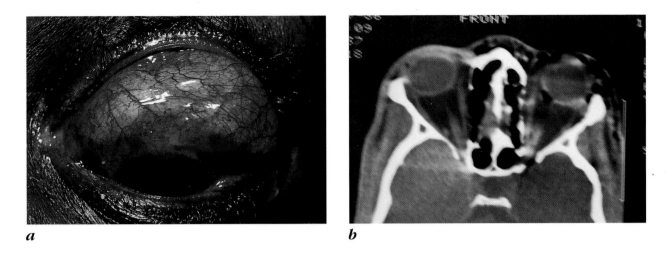

*a*        *b*

**Figure 1.5** *Orbital emphysema secondary to a blunt orbital injury fracturing the medial orbital wall. CT scan demonstrates medial orbital wall fracture and air in orbit (b).*

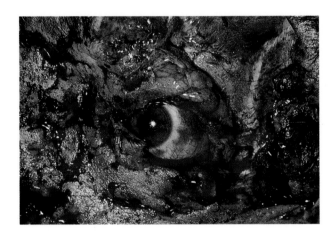

**Figure 1.6** *Automobile accident avulsing both eyelids and brow but completely sparing the globe.*

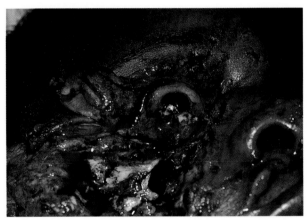

**Figure 1.7** *A similar automobile accident resulting in avulsion of both upper and lower eyelids and disruption of globe.*

degree of vision with modern surgical techniques. It is the practice of the author's team to attempt to save all ruptured globes, especially in less than responsive patients. Often primary repair of globes which are almost certain to have no visual potential is attempted (Fig. 1.8). This reassures the patient that everything possible was done to save the injured eye.

It may also avoid unwanted litigation as the patient accuses the surgeon of removing an eye that might have been saved by a more competent surgeon or claims that vision might have been restored at a more enlightened time. Secondary enucleations are accomplished within 10 days of the injury whenever possible to avoid the rare occurrence of sympathetic

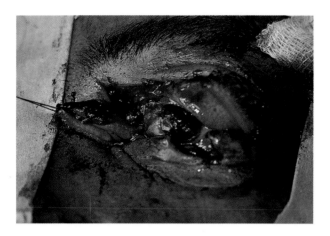

**Figure 1.8** *A broken bottle severely disrupted this globe and eyelids.*

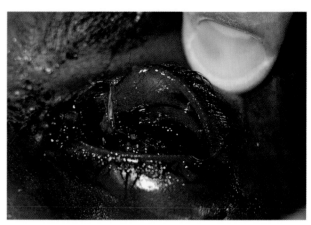

**Figure 1.9** *A gunshot wound completely obliterated this eye. When nothing was found to repair, the globe was primarily enucleated.*

ophthalmia. Patients are offered a second opinion prior to removal of their eye. The only globes that are primarily enucleated are those that are totally destroyed with no hope of obtaining anatomic integrity (Fig. 1.9). These globes will only be removed when the patient is coherent enough to understand the status of their injured eye and give appropriate informed consent.

There is no substitute for a complete eye examination in the patient presenting with periocular trauma (Fig. 1.10). The presence of an obvious eyelid laceration does not mitigate against an occult blunt or penetrating injury to the globe (Fig. 1.10).

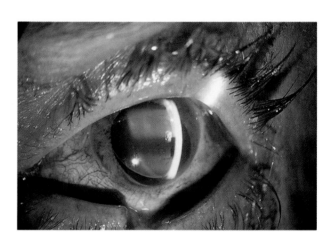

**Figure 1.10** *Slit-lamp examination documents a subluxated lens in this patient referred for repair of an eyelid laceration.*

## INITIAL EVALUATION

How did the injury occur? What was the patient doing, and where were they doing it? Were they striking metal on metal? Or using acids or alkali? If a chemical injury is suspected, irrigate the eyes, and ask questions and examine the patient later.

In all other patient, document visual acuity before examining the patients. The best vision possible under the circumstances of the examination should be obtained. Obviously, in the office or clinic a best-corrected or pinhole vision is desirable and easily obtainable. In the emergency department or at the bedside, a near card is adequate. Remember that older patients will not do so well with a near card unless their presbyopic correction is utilized or they are provided with an appropriate reading aid. A pair of inexpensive +2.5 or +3.0 readers available from most pharmacies is quite convenient to carry along with a near card. Regardless of whether or not a formal eye

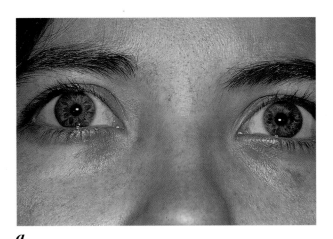

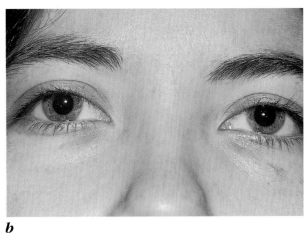

a

b

**Figure 1.11** *Relative afferent pupillary defect. Light is shone into the normal eye (a) and both pupils constrict. When light is shone into the eye with the optic nerve injury, the pupils paradoxically dilate (b).*

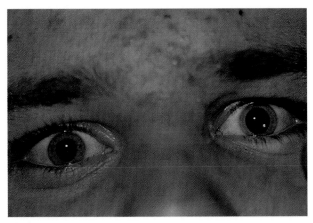

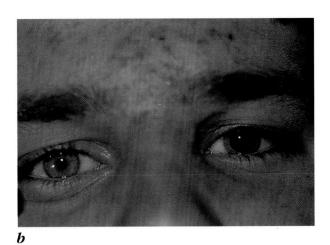

a

b

**Figure 1.12** *Inverse relative afferent pupillary defect. As light is directed into the blind left eye with a dilated pupil, the pupil in the normal right eye dilates. When the light is directed into the normal eye, the pupil constricts briskly (b).*

chart is available, do document visual function. Imagination is required. For example, notations such as 'reads small newsprint at 1 ft,' or 'can count fingers easily at 10 ft' provide sufficient documentation to help obviate a future medicolegal nightmare.

If the visual acuity is not equal and normal, it is imperative to determine why the vision is not the same in both eyes, especially if the worse vision is in the injured eye. A very common mistake is not looking for a relative afferent pupillary defect (RAPD) or an inverse relative afferent pupillary defect prior to dilating the patient's pupils. The RAPD is the *sine qua non* of optic nerve dysfunction. The afferent pupillary defect is the hallmark of an injury in the

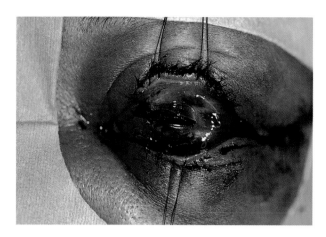

**Figure 1.13** *Obvious corneoscleral laceration caused by blunt trauma.*

anterior portion of the neuro-ophthalmic axis from the ganglion cell layer through the optic disc, through the optic nerve to the lateral geniculate. It is determined by having the patient look at a distant fixation target to avoid near miosis and shining a bright light into the uninjured eye (Fig. 1.11). Both pupils should briskly constrict by the direct and consensual pupil-

lary reactions. The light is then directed into the injured eye. The light is swung from one eye to the other—hence the term 'swinging flashlight test'. If the pupil dilates as the light is directed into it, a RAPD is present, and the examiner should be alerted to the potential for optic nerve injury. Often in the setting of ocular and orbital trauma, the involved pupil may be dilated due to concomitant efferent pupillary dysfunction. When the light is directed into the poorly sighted eye with the dilated pupil, the pupil in the contralateral normal eye dilates. When the light is then directed into the normal eye, the pupil briskly constricts (Fig. 1.12). Although many systems have been designed to grade pupillary responses, the best way to do it is with neutral density camera filters. These filters measure incrementally the amount of light passing through them. They are graded in 0.3 log units. Consequently the examiner can quantify how much injury there is to the anterior neuro-ophthalmic visual axis.

It is very important to shine a light at the same angle into the patient's pupils. After determining whether there is an afferent pupillary defect, it is important to determine if there is some acute media opacity that may be causing the problem. Dense vitreous hemorrhage is often associated with a small afferent pupillary defect.

After visual acuity has been determined and an afferent pupillary defect has been sought, examination can be more narrowly directed. What was the

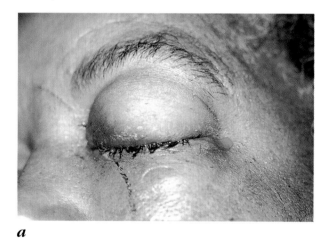

*a*

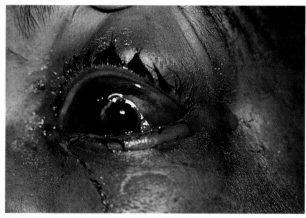

*b*

**Figure 1.14** *Apparent fingernail laceration of the eyelids (a) upon closer examination demonstrates an obvious laceration of the globe (b).*

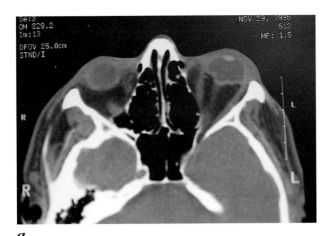

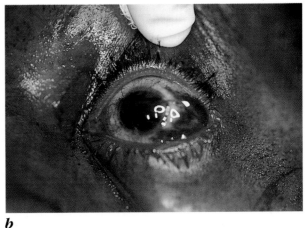

*a*                                           *b*

**Figure 1.15** *CT scan demonstrating obvious posterior collapse of a globe; fundus examination was precluded by a hemorrhage.*

nature of the injury? Is a lacerated globe suspected? If so, a careful slit-lamp examination of the anterior segment is warranted. Look carefully: lacerations of the globe may be obvious (Fig. 1.13) or more occult (Fig. 1.14). Are the cornea, anterior chamber and lens clear? If so, dilate the pupil and carefully examine the lens, vitreous body, fundus and optic nerve. If a good view (or any view) of the fundus is precluded by media opacities, a computed tomography (CT) scan of the eye and orbits may demonstrate disruption of the globe indicative of a rupture or an intraocular foreign body (Fig. 1.15). It is difficult to miss the diagnosis of an obviously ruptured globe if an appropriate, compulsive ocular examination has been performed. Occult ruptures of the globe may prove to be more of a clinical challenge. This is even more important when it is considered that a globe with a small or occult rupture often has excellent visual potential. If the diagnosis is missed or delayed, the eye with excellent visual potential may be blinded by infection or other complications of its injury.

What clinical signs should raise suspicion of an occult rupture of the globe? Evidence for a sharp injury or scratch on the eyelids should alert the clinician that an object may have penetrated the eyelid and lacerated the globe (Fig. 1.14). Decreased vision out of proportion to the apparent injury should prompt the clinician to look hard for an afferent pupillary defect prior to dilating the pupils to rule out the presence of a traumatic optic neuropathy. Excessive conjunctival chemosis or hemorrhage (Fig. 1.16), especially when combined with hypotony of the globe, should alert the clinician to the presence of an occult ruptured globe. An anterior chamber that is deeper on the injured side than on the uninjured should be a cause for suspicion.

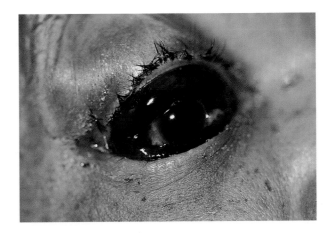

**Figure 1.16** *Hemorrhagic chemosis is very suspicious of an underlying ruptured globe.*

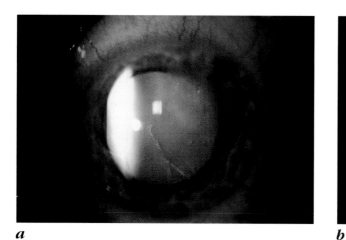

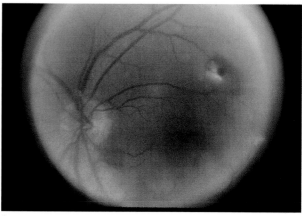

*a*                                                                                        *b*

**Figure 1.17** *Transillumination defects in the iris alerted the clinician to the presence of an intraocular metallic foreign body (b).*

The clinician should be alerted to the possibility of an occult intraocular foreign body by the history of the injury. The classic example is an injury resulting from metal striking metal. The clue may be subtle transillumination defects in the iris tracts in the lens or hemorrhage in the retina (Fig. 1.17). Gonioscopy may demonstrate the foreign body in the anterior chamber angle. Immediate dilatation and thorough examination of the lens, vitreous and fundus may allow detection of the foreign body. If the ocular media is sufficiently opaque to preclude a thorough examination, high-resolution CT scanning or excellent ultrasonography may help detect an intraocular foreign body. Undetected metallic intraocular foreign bodies may be disastrous for the eye shortly after or as a late sequela of trauma. The man in Figure 1.18 was working on his car in a barnyard. He was banging a muffler with a hammer and noted a foreign body sensation in his eye. When it did not resolve in several hours he saw his doctor who gave him some neomycin ointment and told him to see an ophthalmologist in the morning. He arose with a red, painful eye without light perception (Fig. 1.18(a)). A CT scan demonstrated an intraocular metallic foreign body and the stigmata of a panophthalmitis (Fig. 1.18(b)). Vitrectomy was attempted; but rapidly evolved into an evisceration. The foreign body and ocular contents were removed (Fig. 1.18(c)). Cultures confirmed the clinical impression of *Bacillus cereus* endophthalmitis. The clinician should have been alerted to the possibility of an intraocular foreign body by the history of striking metal on metal at the time of the injury and the potential for a devastating infection by the nature of the environment in which the accident occurred.

Several other issues often arise when dealing with an acutely traumatized eye. What is the prognosis for restoring visual function? When should surgery be performed? Does it matter whether it is carried out immediately or delayed for several hours and done electively in the morning or later in the day? What is the role of prophylactic antibiotics? When should an eye be primarily enucleated?

## PROGNOSIS FOR THE RUPTURED GLOBE

In a recent review of 176 ruptured globes,[1] the authors found that a final excellent visual prognosis—defined as visual acuity of 20/60 or better—was correlated with the following manifestations:

1)  An initial visual acuity of 20/200 or better.
2)  A sharp mechanism of injury, that is, a knife or glass wound as opposed to a blunt injury.
3)  A laceration anterior to the recti insertions and measuring less than 10 mm in length.

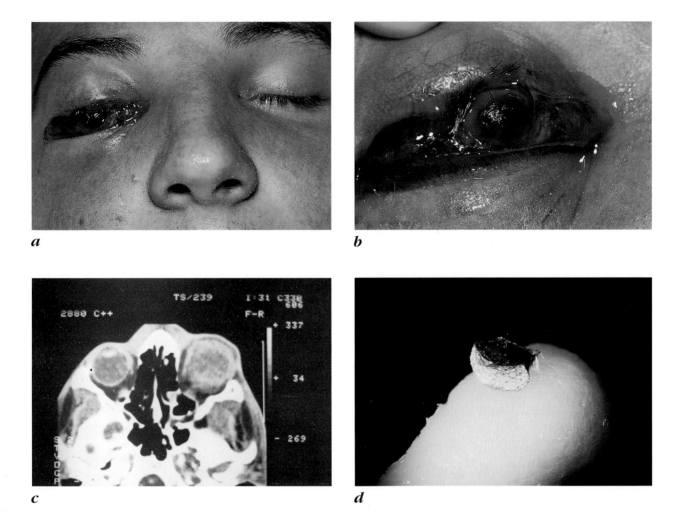

**Figure 1.18** *Patient with* Bacillus cereus *endophthalmitis (a) presenting with a blind, red and painful eye 24 hours after injury (b); CT scan demonstrating diffuse inflammation and a panophthalmitis (c); metallic intraocular foreign body removed at evisceration (d).*

Predictors of poor visual acuity after a ruptured globe not surprisingly included:

1) An initial visual acuity of no light perception (NLP) or light perception (LP) only.
2) A blunt mechanism of injury or an injury caused by a missile or a projectile.
3) Lacerations measuring more than 10 mm in length and extending posterior to the plane of insertion of the recti muscles.

This represents statistical confirmation of what we have intuitively known for many years: globes with small anterior lacerations made by sharp instruments and presenting with good visual acuity do well (Fig. 1.19). Globes suffering more severe injury do not often do well (Fig. 1.20).

## PROPHYLACTIC ANTIBIOTICS

Use or abuse of prophylactic antibiotics has been argued in the literature since antibiotics became routinely available to the practicing surgeon.

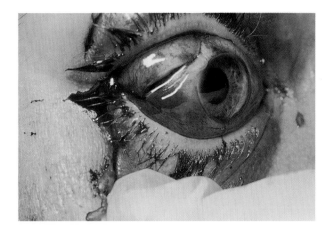

**Figure 1.19** *An anterior scleral laceration caused by a sharp instrument has a good visual prognosis.*

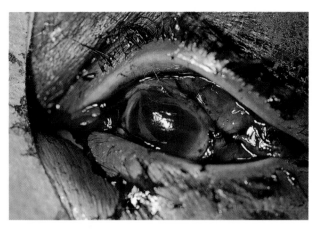

**Figure 1.20** *Large posterior lacerations caused by blunt trauma have a poor visual prognosis.*

Ophthalmology is no different, and arguments can be, and often are, made passionately and not backed by any reasonable data either advocating their use or chastising the poor house officer who had the temerity to use them. One recent study puts the issue in perspective and provides a reasonable rationale for the use of prophylactic antibiotics in patients with ruptured globes. Arivasu,[2] citing the poor diagnosis of post-traumatic endophthalmitis, cultured the anterior chambers of patients with ruptured globes. Patients either received intravenous antibiotics or did not. One-third of the patients who had positive bacterial cultures from their anterior chamber at the time of surgery had antibiotic therapy. Patients receiving preoperative intravenous antibiotics had a markedly reduced incidence of positive bacterial cultures from their anterior chamber at the time of surgery compared with those patients not receiving preoperative antibiotics. The differences were very significant ($P = 0.002$). The authors conclude that this decreased incidence in intraocular bacterial contamination leads to a decreased risk of postoperative endophthalmitis. The timing and duration of administration of the antibiotic used has little bearing upon the final results. The essence is that prophylactic antibiotics decrease intraocular bacterial contamination in ruptured globes. If it is believed that less bacterial contamination leads to a lesser incidence of postoperative endophthalmitis, then prophylactic intravenous antibiotics should be used prior to repairing a ruptured globe. Either cephazolin, vancomycin or ciprofloxacin will provide adequate gram-positive coverage. Vancomycin should be used if there is concern specifically about a *Bacillus* species infection (Fig. 1.18). If there is concern about mixed gram-positive and gram-negative contamination, additional gram-negative coverage may be added. Ceftazidime or amikacin may provide excellent coverage of gram-negative organisms. The following antibiotic regimens may be used for prevention of endophthalmitis:

1) Vancomycin 1 g intravenously every 12 hours: provides excellent gram-positive coverage and is especially effective against *Bacillus* spp. and *Staphylococcus*, the two most common gram-positive organisms causing post-traumatic intraocular infections.
2) Ceftazidime 1 g intravenously every 12 hours: provides excellent gram-negative coverage.
3) Ciprofloxacin 750 mg orally every 12 hours: may be substituted for vancomycin but may not be active against *Streptococcus*.
4) Amikacin 1 g intravenously every 12 hours: may be substituted for ceftazidime for gram-negative coverage.

## TIMING OF SURGERY

Several studies have demonstrated that there is no difference in visual outcome in patients undergoing immediate repair of their ruptured globes and those waiting up to 24 hours.[3] The author advocates waiting until the patient has been cleared for general anesthesia by the other services involved in their care, has undergone appropriate imaging studies to detect concurrent injury to adjacent structures (brain and sinuses), and has received preoperative antibiotics. Depending on the degree of injury and the complexity of the surgery involved, a competent operating-room staff familiar with ophthalmic surgical procedures varies from a luxury to an absolute necessity to render adequate patient care. It is no crime to wait a few hours for more experienced personnel to be available in the operating room.

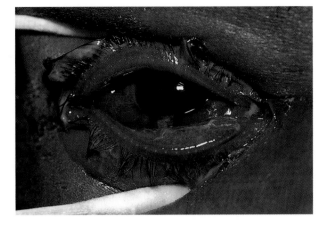

**Figure 1.21** *Acute purulent gonococcal conjunctivitis.*

## THE RED EYE

The patient presenting with a red eye may manifest a wide range of ophthalmologic and neurologic pathology, ranging from a simple subconjunctival hemorrhage to an occult rupture of the globe, or from simple conjunctivitis to a carotid-cavernous fistula. As with many other ophthalmologic disorders, a brief history and careful examination often result in an accurate diagnosis. What were you doing when you noticed that your eye was red? The ramifications of awakening with a painless red eye (conjunctivitis or subconjunctival hemorrhage) are very different from noticing a painful eye after scraping rust from metal (corneal foreign body) or a painful red eye with decreased vision after hammering metal on metal (intraocular foreign body). The index of suspicion for endophthalmitis is always raised if there is a history of antecedent intraocular surgery, even in the somewhat remote past. An early endophthalmitis by a relatively nonvirulent organism may present as a smoldering red eye after cataract surgery. Early diagnosis and treatment may be sight-saving.

Patients with iritis may present with a painful red eye. This pain will not be relieved with the administration of a topical anesthetic as will the pain patients suffer from corneal abrasions of foreign bodies. The flare and cell in the anterior chamber should be evident, but not always obvious, on slit-lamp examination.

Acute angle-closure glaucoma often presents as a painful red eye. The pupil may be fixed and mid-dilated. Iritis and a shallow anterior chamber are evident on slit-lamp examination. The diagnosis is confirmed by markedly elevated intraocular pressure.

Orbital inflammation predominantly affecting the anterior orbit and extraocular muscles may present as a very painful eye with a normal-appearing cornea and no evidence for iritis.

Patients with carotid-cavernous fistulas may present with an acute onset of pain accompanied by decreased vision or diplopia. These globes are often proposed, and it may be difficult to differentiate them from severe orbital inflammatory disease or cellulitis.

## CONJUNCTIVITIS

Most clinicians think of conjunctivitis when confronted with a red eye. Most conjunctivitis, whether viral, bacterial or allergic, are self-limiting, will resolve with or without treatment, and are rarely visually threatening. The exception is acute purulent gonococcal conjunctivitis (Fig. 1.21). Since the gonococcus microorganism can penetrate intact corneal epithelium and cause loss of the eye, this a true ophthalmologic emergency. Diagnosis is confirmed by noting gram-negative intracellular diplococci on examination of a smear of the purulent discharge. Treatment consists of irrigating the purulent material from the eye and application of appropriate topical and intravenous antibiotics. Topical antimicrobial agents alone are ineffective in treating gonococcal keratoconjunctivitis. The

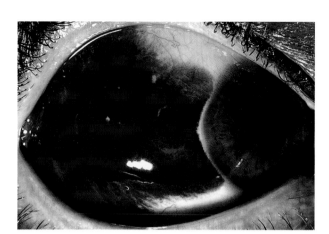

**Figure 1.22** *Subconjunctival hemorrhage caused by a broken blood vessel.*

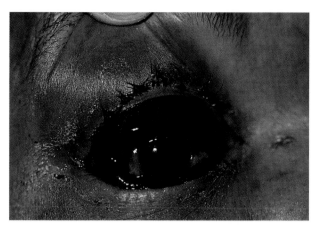

**Figure 1.23** *Excessive subconjunctival hemorrhagic chemosis should alert the clinician to the presence of a ruptured globe.*

mainstay of topical therapy is copious irrigation of the involved eye with sterile saline solution to wash away the bacterial toxins. This may need to be done initially every hour. Topical gentamycin, erythromycin or bacitracin may be used four to six times daily. Topical therapy alone is inadequate. Systemic therapy is essential. Patients with kerato-conjunctivitis should be hospitalized and treated with intravenous ceftriaxone, 1 g twice daily. Penicillin-allergic patients may be treated with spectinomycin 2 g intramuscularly (IM) twice daily. Either treatment should continue for 3–5 days.

## SUBCONJUNCTIVAL HEMORRHAGE

Subconjunctival hemorrhages are almost always benign, caused by a broken subconjunctival blood vessel (Fig. 1.22). These patients often present to the emergency room or to the ophthalmologist's office concerned by the appearance of so much blood around their eyes. A history of blunt or possibly penetrating intraocular trauma should be elicited. Excessive chemosis accompanying a subconjunctival hemorrhage should alert the clinician to a possible occult rupture of the globe (Fig. 1.23). Hemorrhage and subconjunctival emphysema should prompt detection of an occult or obvious medial orbital wall

fracture (Fig. 1.24). Patients with medial orbital wall fractures may be treated with oral antibiotics, that is, cephalexin 500 mg four times daily for one week, to prevent orbital infection. The vast majority of patients with subconjunctival hemorrhages can be reassured after a complete, careful examination of their eyes that they are fine and that the blood will reabsorb within several weeks.

## CORNEAL FOREIGN BODY/ABRASION

Corneal abrasions are one of the most common reasons that patients visit any physician, be it an ophthalmologist or an emergency room physician. Although common, and often rapidly self-healing, an infected corneal ulcer may develop (Fig. 1.25). Intact corneal epithelium is only penetrable by two bacteria: the Neisseria gonococcus microorganism and *Corynebacterium diphtheriae*. Once the epithelium is violated by abrasion, scratch or foreign body, it becomes susceptible to a plethora of microorganisms. Corneal epithelial defects heal rapidly, usually within 24–48 hours. Little can be done to enhance the healing process. The role of the physician is to control pain and prevent infection.

A corneal foreign body or abrasion should be evident on the slit-lamp examination. A corneal

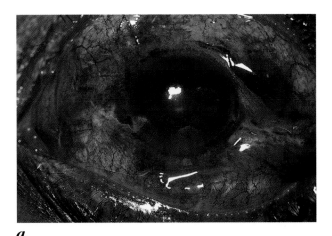

*a*

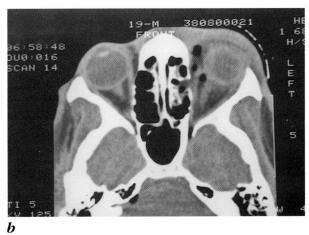

*b*

**Figure 1.24** *Conjunctival chemosis and emphysema. CT scan demonstrating a medial orbital wall fracture and orbital emphysema (b).*

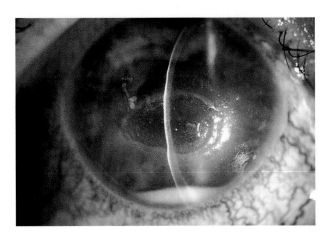

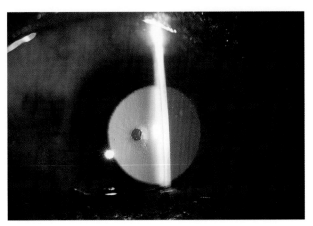

**Figure 1.25** *Corneal ulcer and hypopyon secondary to infected corneal abrasion.*

**Figure 1.26** *Corneal foreign body.*

foreign body is usually obvious (Fig. 1.26), but a subtle corneal abrasion may be missed unless the cornea is stained with a 2% sodium fluorescein solution (Fig. 1.27). Placing a drop of topical anesthetic in the eye should almost immediately relieve the pain of a corneal abrasion or foreign body. This may be done diagnostically but never therapeutically.

It is important to detect a foreign body under the eyelid or hidden in the upper fornix. Linear scratches on the cornea are usually diagnostic (Fig. 1.28). Once these scratches are detected, the clinician must be certain that there is no residual foreign body under the upper eyelid or in the fornix. Double eversion of the eyelid may be necessary, and such foreign bodies

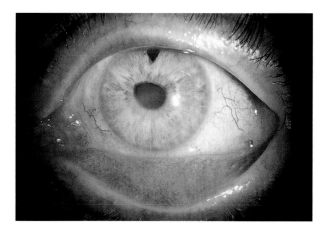

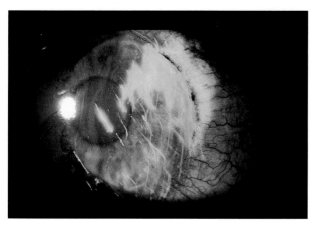

**Figure 1.27** *Subtle corneal abrasion detected with fluorescein stain.*

**Figure 1.28** *Linear corneal abrasions caused by a foreign body under the upper eyelid.*

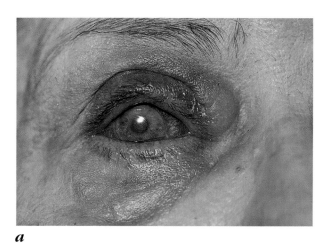

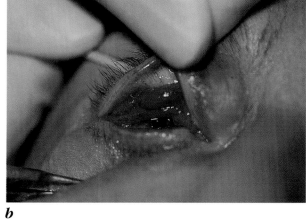

*a*

*b*

**Figure 1.29** *Patient with a corneal erosion refractory to treatment. Double eversion of the eyelid detects an occult foreign body causing recurrent refractory corneal erosion (b).*

may be elusive (Fig. 1.29). Double eversion is accomplished by first everting the eyelid over a cotton-tipped applicator and subsequently placing a DesMarres retractor (Storz Instruments, St Louis, MI) under the folded tarsus and retracting superiorly, exposing the upper fornix (Fig. 1.29). If a DesMarres retractor is not available, a paperclip can be bent at right angles to accomplish the same purpose.

Antibiotic drops or ointment are the mainstays of treatment. Some argue that ointments interfere with the epithelial healing process, but this is probably not true. Ointments have a longer contact time with the cornea and are probably more reliable than drops.

There is also the 'to patch or not to patch' debate. Proponents of a tight pressure patch state that keeping the eye tightly closed provides immediate

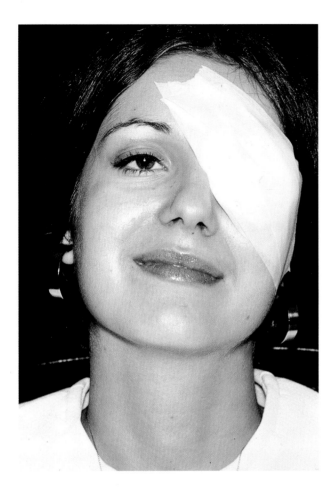

**Figure 1.30** *A properly placed pressure patch immobilizes the eyelids but allows the patient to smile and masticate.*

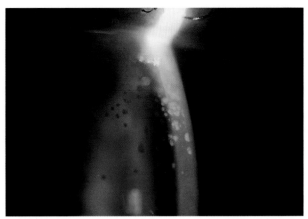

**Figure 1.31** *Recalcitrant iritis as a manifestation of an occult intraocular foreign body.*

symptomatic relief and by immobilizing the eyelid does not interfere with the healing epithelium. Patching is a well accepted standard of care, but must be approached with some caveats. First, a patch must be placed properly (Fig. 1.30). A properly placed patch will close the eye, immobilize the eyelid and still allow the patient to smile and masticate (Fig. 1.30). A poorly placed patch is worse than no treatment at all. There are several arguments against patching. It may increase the chance of infection by increasing the temperature in the conjunctival cul-de-sac and promoting the growth of bacteria. The duration of action of an antibiotic ointment is 3 hours. A patched eye therefore is only protected by the antibiotic for 3 hours. The eye is subsequently unprotected. Since most patches are placed overnight, there is theoretically a good deal of time when the patched eye is more susceptible to infection. In one study, patients with contact-lens abrasions that were patched were more likely to develop severe *Pseudomonas* ulcers than those that were not patched.[4] Another, more recent study describes more rapid healing and less pain in patients who were not patched as opposed to patients who were patched. A corollary study found that if nonsteroidal anti-inflammatory drops were added, pain was almost completely eliminated in the no-patch group.[5,6] These abrasions were less than 1 cm$^2$. There was no statistically significant data for larger abrasions. Patching relieves pain in patients with large abrasions and may well be of benefit. Regardless of whether a patient is treated with patching, antibiotic ointment or drops, careful daily follow-up is essential until the abrasion is healed to detect and treat any incipient corneal infection.[7]

## INTRAOCULAR FOREIGN BODY

An occult intraocular foreign body can present as recurrent ocular irritation accompanied by a mild to severe iritis (Fig. 1.31), developing into a fulminant endophthalmitis. An appropriate history is very

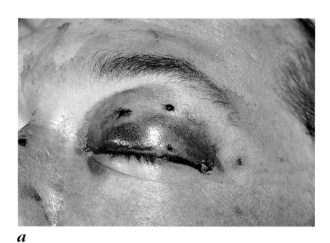
*a*

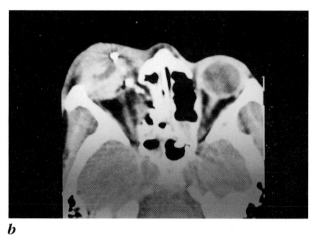
*b*

**Figure 1.32** *Swollen lids obviating a careful eye examination in a patient with a gunshot wound to the face (a). CT scan demonstrating ruptured globe and intraocular pellets (b).*

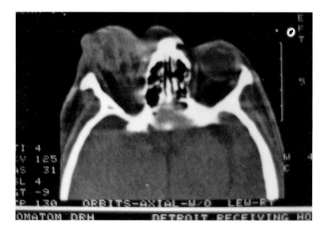

**Figure 1.33** *CT scan demonstrating a ruptured globe in a patient difficult to examine due to excessive lid swelling and chemosis.*

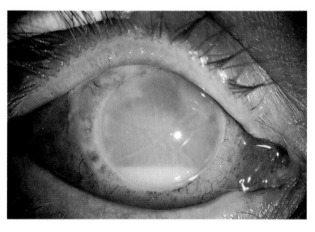

**Figure 1.34** *Early bacterial endophthalmitis manifesting cloudy media and hypopyon.*

helpful in establishing the diagnosis early. Examination of the anterior chamber angle by gonioscopy may be very helpful in detecting an occult foreign body in the anterior chamber of a patient with recalcitrant iritis or unexplained hyphema. Detection of an intraocular foreign body is essential if proper management decisions are to be made. High-resolution CT scanning of patients with periocular trauma and cloudy media may be very helpful in diagnosing occult foreign bodies or ruptured globes (Figs 1.32 and 1.33).

Early diagnosis of an intraocular foreign body plays an important role in preventing the development of endophthalmitis. Eyes with intraocular foreign bodies detected within 24 hours of injury have a 3.5% incidence of endophthalmitis. The incidence

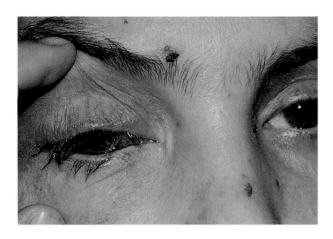

**Figure 1.35** *Patient with early endophthalmitis secondary to a penetrating injury.*

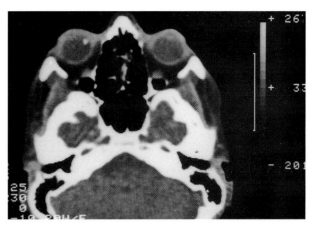

**Figure 1.36** *CT scan demonstrating retrolental bony density.*

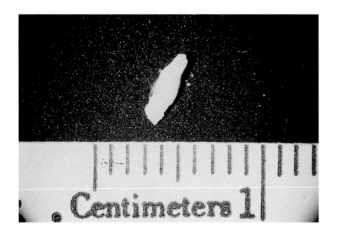

**Figure 1.37** *Osseous foreign body visualized in Fig. 1.36 removed at vitrectomy.*

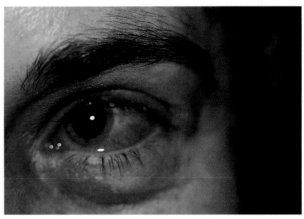

**Figure 1.38** *Angle-closure glaucoma.*

increases to 13.4% for eyes with foreign bodies detected more than 24 hours after injury.[8]

## ENDOPHTHALMITIS

Bacterial endophthalmitis should be considered in any patient with recent intraocular surgery present-

ing with a red eye. If the patient complains of increased floaters, blurry vision or pain, consider the diagnosis to be endophthalmitis until proven otherwise (Fig. 1.34). Especially with today's small-incision cataract surgery, patients might notice decreased vision as an early sign, especially if the infection is caused by a relatively nonvirulent organism. Early diagnosis is important, because these

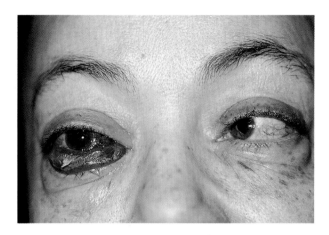

**Figure 1.39** *A red eye and inflamed orbit due to periscleritis.*

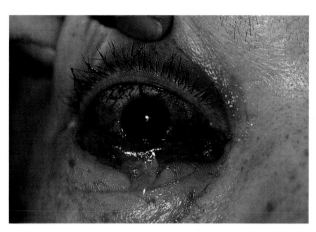

**Figure 1.40** *Proptosis, sixth nerve palsy, and arterialization of conjunctival vessels are telltale signs of a carotid-cavernous fistula.*

patients are the ones most likely to benefit by early therapeutic intervention.

Diagnosing an intraocular infection with no history of antecedent surgery or obvious trauma is more difficult. Suspicion, and a good history and examination are the keys to early diagnosis and treatment. A 19-year-old girl was arguing with her boyfriend, who was distraught. He put a revolver to his jaw and threatened to shoot himself unless she would marry him. She refused, and he shot himself and was taken to hospital. The girl went home and, several hours later, noticed a foreign-body sensation in her right eye. She went to the emergency room and was told that she had conjunctivitis, was given an antibiotic drop, and sent home. The next day she noted pain in the eye and returned to the emergency room. This time an iritis was diagnosed and she was treated with cycloplegic drops and topical steroids. The next day, while visiting her now more distraught boyfriend at the county hospital, she was seen by the resident on call, who noted significant intraocular inflammation, cloudy media and decreased vision (Fig. 1.35). A CT scan was obtained, and a small bony density was evident just behind the lens (Fig. 1.36). At vitrectomy, this proved to be bone (Fig. 1.37) compatible with her boyfriend's demolished mandible. After a course of intravitreal and intravenous antibiotics, normal visual function was restored.

Appropriate history and a careful examination of the eye would have expedited the diagnosis of an intraocular foreign body in this patient. Any patient presenting with an acute onset red eye or foreign-body sensation should be questioned, looking for a story compatible with penetration of the eye by a high-speed projectile—in this case, a fragment of bone, but classically an intraocular metallic foreign body caused by a metal-striking-metal injury.

A 38-year-old man was striking a nail with a hammer and noted a foreign-body sensation in his left eye. He presented to the clinic and the metal-on-metal history alerted the examiner to examine the eye carefully for evidence of occult intraocular penetration. A transillumination defect in the iris (Fig. 1.16) prompted careful fundus examination and the intraocular foreign body was detected and appropriate treatment was instituted (see Chapter 5).

## IRITIS

Patients with iritis present with pain and photophobia. Discomfort is not relieved with topical anesthetics. Intraocular pressure may be elevated or relatively decreased. Flare and cells are visible in the anterior chamber on slit-lamp examination. The pupil may be miotic or irregular due to posterior synechiae. Treatment consists of dilatation and cycloplegia of the pupil, topical steroids, and control of intraocular pressure as necessary.

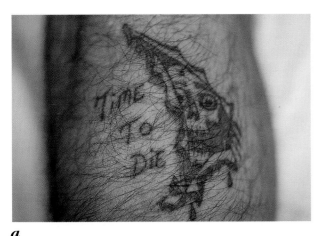

*a*

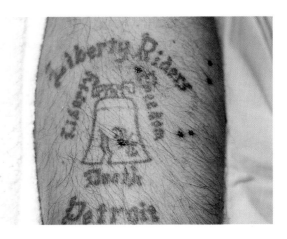

*b*

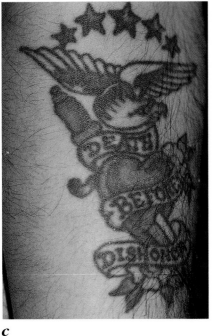

*c*

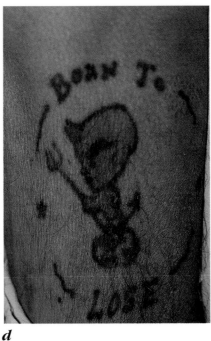

*d*

**Figure 1.41** *Telltale tattoos often adorn patients with self-destructive personalities who are prone to injury ((a)–(d)).*

## ANGLE-CLOSURE GLAUCOMA

Patients with angle-closure glaucoma present with a painful red eye and a mid-dilated fixed pupil (Fig. 1.38). Pain is often extreme and may be accompanied by nausea and vomiting. Intraocular pressure is markedly elevated. Treatment consists of lowering the intraocular pressure with miotic agents and hyperosmotics and performing a laser iridotomy to break the attack and prevent it from recurring.

## THE INFLAMED ORBIT (THE RED ORBIT)

The differential diagnosis of the inflamed orbit (Fig. 1.39) includes orbital cellulitis (pre- and postseptal), idiopathic orbital inflammation (pseudotumor), acute dysthyroid orbitopathy and carotid-cavernous fistula. These entities can usually be differentiated after examining the patient and obtaining a CT scan and will be discussed in detail in Chapter 9.

## CAROTID-CAVERNOUS FISTULA

A carotid-cavernous fistula is a communication between the carotid artery, or an arteriole in the cavernous sinus, and the cavernous sinus. The subsequent high-flow to low-flow state causes the characteristic signs and symptoms including proptosis, conjunctival infection, and an audible bruit. Diplopia often occurs and is most commonly due to a sixth-nerve palsy (Fig. 1.40). Carotid-cavernous fistulas often occur after trauma, but may occur spontaneously. CT scans demonstrate enlargement of the superior ophthalmic vein and extraocular muscles. Recognition of the characteristic signs and symptoms with compatible CT findings should prompt cerebral angiography for definitive diagnosis.

## SPECIAL CONSIDERATIONS IN OCULAR TRAUMA

Patients suffering ocular trauma may be divided into two types—those individuals who have had an accident, be it sports-, work- or automobile-related, and those with self-destructive personalities. The former make up the majority of normal patients. They lead active lives, and when an accident occurs it is very disruptive to their lifestyle. Prevention and education are the keys to diminishing the incidence of ocular and adnexal injuries in these patients. Patients should be instructed on the use of safety glasses at work and at play. Most workplaces mandate the use of safety glass on the job, but accidents still occur when patients are injured while working at home and not wearing their glasses. Participants in racquet sports are prone to ocular injury, as are skiers. The author instructs his skiing patients to use Gargoyle glasses (Gargoyles Inc., Kent, Washington) from the moment they leave the lodge to the time they return from the slopes. Many ski-related ocular injuries result from a misguided ski pole while waiting on line or walking to the slopes. Gargoyles are also excellent for racquet sports and come in a variety of shades from clear to mirrored. Gargoyles, or any safety glasses, should be 3 mm-thick polycarbonate and have reinforced temples so that they will not shatter when struck. One-eyed patients should be instructed to keep something, that is, safety glasses, between their eyes and their environment at all times.

It is important to detect patients with self-destructive personalities. They are often victims of many separate injuries, sometimes self-inflicted and sometimes bestowed upon them by others. Patients with these personality types are often decorated with a variety of tattoo adornments (Fig. 1.41). The author calls it the 'born to love/born to lose' syndrome. It is important to identify these personality types, for they may be very unreliable and quite litigious.

## REFERENCES

1 Esmaeli B, Elner S, Schork A, Elner V. Predictive factors for the ruptured globe. Visual outcome and ocular survival after penetrating trauma. *Ophthalmology* 1995; **102**: 393–400.

2 Arivasu RG. The value of prophylactic intravenous antibiotics in patients with ruptured globes. *Am J Ophthalmol* 1995; **119**: 181–8.

3 Barr CC. Prognostic factors in corneoscleral lacerations. *Arch Ophthalmol* 1983; **101**: 919–24.

4 Clemens CS, Cohen EJ, Arentsen JJ et al. Pseudomonas ulcers following patching of corneal abrasions associated with contact lens wear. *CLAO* 1987; **13**: 161–3.

5 Kaiser PKA. Comparison of pressure patching and no patching for corneal abrasion due to foreign body removal. *Ophthalmology* 1995; **102**: 1936–42.

6 Abelson MB. The finer points of corneal abrasion management. *Rev Ophthalmol* 1995; **(Feb)**: 111–12.

7 McLeod SD, LaBree D, Tayyanipour R, et al. The importance of initial management in the treatment of severe infectious corneal ulcers. *Ophthalmology* 1995; **102**: 1443–8.

8 Thompson JT, Paarver LM, Enger C and National Eye Trauma Study (NETS). Endophthalmitis after penetrating ocular injuries with retained intraocular foreign bodies. *Ophthalmology* 1993; **100**: 1468–74.

## Chapter 2 The ruptured globe

As mentioned in Chapter 1, the ruptured globe is a relative ophthalmologic emergency. There have been numerous studies seeking to facilitate the diagnosis of the ruptured globe and to predict which injured globes are more likely to yield functional vision after repair.[1-3] Recently reviewing 176 ruptured globes, Esmaeli et al.[4] found the following to be predictors of attaining a visual acuity of 20/60 or better after suffering a ruptured globe: an initial visual acuity of 20/200 or better; location of the wound anterior to the insertion of the recti muscles; a wound length of 10 mm or smaller; and a sharp mechanism of injury. Figure 2.1 demonstrates this type of injury. Visual acuity was 20/100, and the wound was small and anterior.

Predictors of a poor visual prognosis are an initial visual acuity of light perception to no light perception; wounds greater than 10 mm in length; wounds located posterior to the plane of the recti muscles; and those wounds caused by blunt or missile injury.

Figure 2.2 demonstrates a ruptured globe with a very poor prognosis for useful vision. The injury is large, posterior and the initial visual acuity is very poor.

In essence, small anterior lacerations made by sharp objects have a good visual prognosis, while large posterior lacerations resulting from blunt trauma have a much poorer prognosis.

There are no firm guidelines for timing repair of a ruptured globe. Most authorities agree that repair should be done within 24 hours. There is no difference in visual prognosis between those patients repaired immediately and those repaired within 24 hours of injury.[5] There is no great advantage to immediate repair if either operating room, patient or surgeon are not prepared for the procedure. It is of no advantage to operate upon a patient with a stomach full of food and drink and risk possible aspiration and other potential anesthetic complications if comparable results can be obtained by

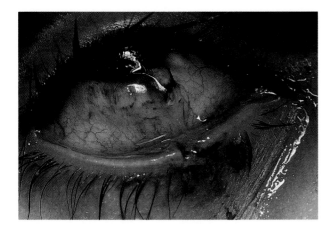

**Figure 2.1** *A small anterior scleral wound inflicted in a knife fight has a good visual prognosis.*

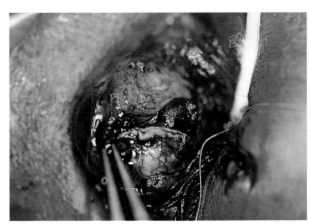

**Figure 2.2** *A large posterior scleral rupture secondary to blunt trauma has a poor visual prognosis.*

waiting until the patient is better prepared for surgery.[5] There is an increased incidence of postoperative endophthalmitis in patients repaired more than 24 hours after injury.[6,7]

Should intravenous prophylactic antibiotics be used? Probably yes. Studies have demonstrated[8] that treatment with intravenous prophylactic antibiotics decreases bacterial colonization of aqueous humor cultured at the time of surgical repair. Treatment with broad spectrum intravenous antibiotics decreases the risk of postoperative traumatic endophthalmitis by decreasing the incidence of intraocular microbial contamination. The incidence of bacterial contamination was over 30% of ruptured globes studied. The time to treatment and the duration of antibiotic therapy prior to surgery were not significant. An antibiotic regimen consisting of 1 g vancomycin and 1 g cephtazidime every 12 hours begun prior to surgery and continued for a total of 40 hours should provide coverage for most common organisms. Continuing prophylactic antibiotics for more than 48 hours is not necessary and increases the possibility of selecting resistant organisms.

The patient is ready for surgery, the intravenous antibiotics have been given, and general anesthesia is being induced. Although most ophthalmologists consider it general knowledge, it is wise to remind the anesthesia personnel that you are dealing with a ruptured globe and to avoid depolarizing agents like succinyl choline that may cause a tetanic contraction of the recti muscles, expressing the ocular contents and converting a salvageable eye into an operative disaster (Fig. 2.3).

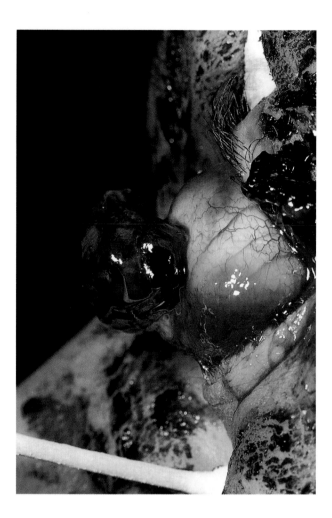

**Figure 2.3** *Expulsion of intraocular contents due to tetanic contraction of extraocular muscles.*

## OPERATIVE TECHNIQUE

Under general anesthesia, the uninvolved eye is routinely taped and shielded to protect it from any accidental injury. The operative site (not the ruptured globe) is carefully prepared with Betadine solution (Purdue–Frederick, Norwalk, CT). If the orbit is swollen, a lateral canthotomy is performed and the eyelids are separated with 4-0 silk traction sutures placed in the upper and lower lids. This prevents excessive pressure being applied to the globe by an eyelid speculum and allows separation of the lids in a controlled fashion. A 360° peritomy is performed and hemostasis obtained with a wet-field and bipolar cautery. Relaxing incisions are made in each quadrant. A double-armed, 6-0 Vicryl suture may be

placed in each of the four pieces of conjunctiva and clipped to the drapes. This retracts the conjunctiva and allows excellent exposure. Tenon's capsule is then excised from the conjunctiva back to the extraocular muscle insertions (Fig. 2.4).

The injury is inspected with magnification and illumination provided by the operating microscope. Uveal tissue prolapsing from a sceral laceration (Fig. 2.5) can be gently teased back into the eye using a fine cannula and a viscoelastic solution. A 7-0 Vicryl suture may then be placed through each side of the laceration and repair begun. If the uveal tissue continues to prolapse, it can be reposited with more viscoelastic. Suturing continues until the wound is closed (Fig. 2.6). A more posterior scleral laceration is more difficult to close. These posterior lacerations are more efficiently closed with loupe magnification instead of the operating microscope. Exposure may

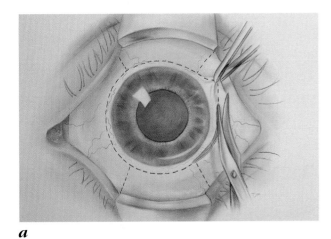

*a*

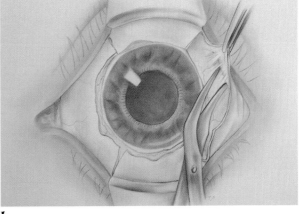

*b*

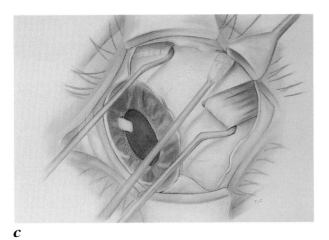

*c*

**Figure 2.4** *Peritomy is performed 360° (a), relaxing incisions are made in each quadrant (b) and the extraocular muscle insertions are exposed (c).*

be quite difficult, and orbital retraction techniques utilizing the DesMarres and malleable retractors may facilitate exposure. After the laceration is identified, a suture may be placed, closing its most anterior aspect. This suture may be left long and utilized to apply forward traction gently on the globe to facilitate exposure of the more posterior aspects of the laceration (Fig. 2.6). It is essential to obtain excellent exposure of the posterior extent of a scleral laceration. These lacerations, especially if the result of blunt trauma, have a tendency to be hidden under the recti muscles where the sclera is thinnest. If this is suspected, the muscle should be sutured as for a recession and severed from the globe (Fig. 2.7). After the laceration is sutured, the muscle may then be reattached to the site of its original insertion. It is important to look routinely under each muscle to search for occult lacerations. This can be

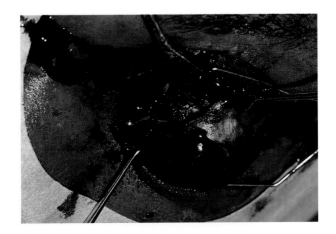

**Figure 2.5** *Scleral laceration with uveal prolapse. Exposure enhanced using DesMarres retractor and muscle-hooks.*

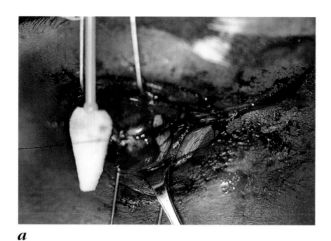

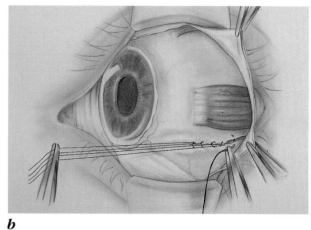

*a*  *b*

**Figure 2.6** *Hand-over-hand technique for repairing a posterior scleral laceration. Exposure is facilitated with a DesMarres retractor.*

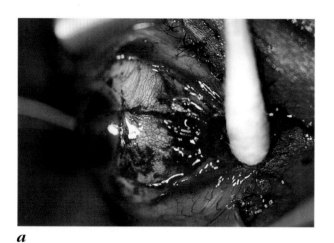

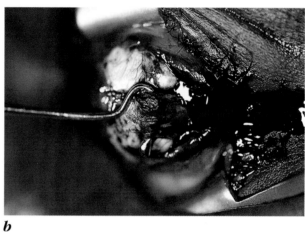

*a*  *b*

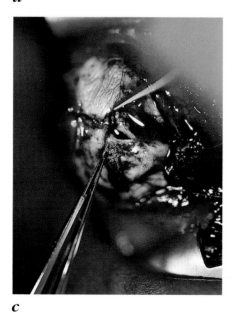

*c*

**Figure 2.7** *Scleral laceration (a) extending to the lateral rectus muscle (b). Large posterior laceration evident (c) after disinsertion of the muscle.*

accomplished using two muscle-hooks and a cotton-tipped applicator to manipulate the globe and the extraocular muscle (Fig. 2.4(c)). Each quadrant of the globe should be carefully explored using a cotton-tipped applicator for hemostasis and to manipulate tissue gently. After the globe is explored and the laceration sutured, the conjunctiva is closed with the previously placed 6-0 or 7-0 Vicryl sutures. To repair

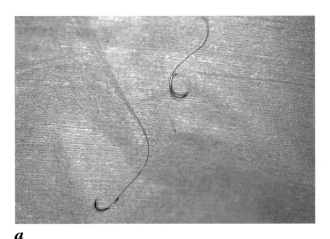

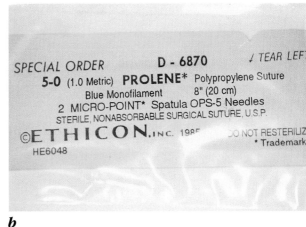

*a*                                                          *b*

**Figure 2.8** *OPS needle on a 5-0 Prolene suture. Curvature and strength of this needle make it ideal for reinserting the lateral canthal structures to the lateral orbital wall.*

the lateral canthotomy, a double-armed 5-0 Prolene suture with an OPS needle (Fig. 2.8) is placed through the upper and lower lateral canthal tendon remnants and tarsus, and both arms of the suture are placed through the periosteum at the inner aspect of the lateral orbital wall at the level of the pupil. This reapproximates the lateral canthal angle and places the lids snugly against the globe.

## CORNEAL-SCLERAL LACERATION

A corneal-scleral laceration (Fig. 2.9) is approached in a similar fashion. Wounds that cross the limbus are reapproximated with 7-0 Vicryl sutures. After the limbal wounds are approximated, the cornea is repaired with 10-0 nylon interrupted sutures. The wound is halved with 10-0 nylon suture and uvea reposited using a cyclodialysis spatula or a viscoelastic. The wound is then halved again and uvea again reposited (Fig. 2.10). This is continued until a water-tight closure is obtained. The anterior chamber is reformed with a viscoelastic, and the sutures are buried. If the sutures are tied with an initial double knot followed by two single knots, the resultant knot should be buried in the suture tract. This gently enhances patient comfort during the long postopera-

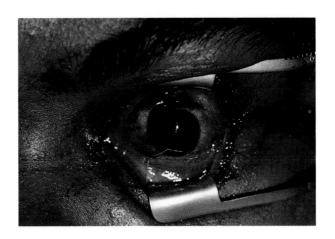

**Figure 2.9** *Corneal-scleral laceration.*

tive period. The corneal wound is then checked for leaks with a 2% fluorescein solution. A paracentesis wound is made at the limbus with a superblade, and iris is swept away from the wounds with a cyclo-dialysis spatula or viscoelastic and a cannula. The scleral portion of the wound may be closed with a 7-0 Vicryl or equivalent suture. Prolapsed uvea is cultured, and the surgeon must decide what uvea to

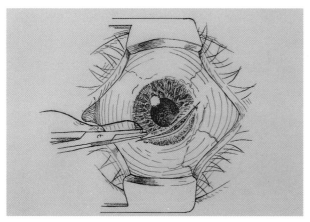

*a*

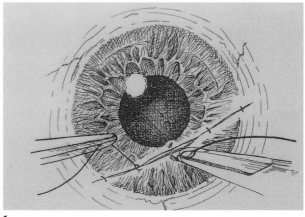

*b*

**Figure 2.10** *Repair sequence for corneal-scleral laceration. The corneoscleral limbus is approximated with a 7-0 Vicryl suture (a). The corneal laceration is approximated utilizing 10-0 nylon sutures. The halving technique closes half of the open incision with each suture (b).*

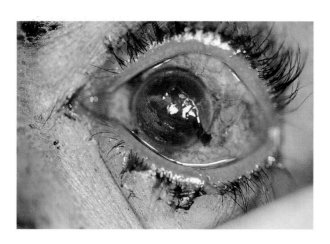

**Figure 2.11** *Corneal laceration with prolapsed iris.*

reposit and what uvea to excise. If the uvea is necrotic, contaminated or incarcerated for more than 24 hours it should be excised. If it is not necrotic, as much of the uvea as possible should be reposited. Prolapsing uvea may be managed with viscoelastic which may also be used to reform and maintain the anterior chamber during surgery.

## CORNEAL LACERATION

A pure corneal laceration (Fig 2.11) should be repaired with 10-0 nylon sutures with buried knots. Sutures should be passed either through full-thickness cornea or to the level of Descemet's membrane. More shallow passage of sutures will result in posterior wound gape and adherent leukomas (Fig. 2.12). The edges should be well approximated; however, the sutures should not be too tight for they may induce a large amount of astigmatism. The visual axis should be avoided with the needle tract. One should endeavor not to place a suture within the 2 mm pupillary axis, for it will exacerbate scarring and decrease visual function.

## COMPLICATED CORNEAL LACERATIONS

Large stellate corneal lacerations or those with significant loss of tissue may tax the ingenuity of the most experienced surgeon (Fig. 2.13). Excessive astigmatism is not a concern in these patients. The surgeon is trying to maintain the integrity of the eye, realizing that a penetrating keratoplasty or refractive procedure will be necessary in the future. Large stellate

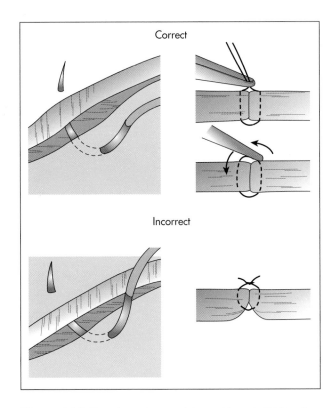

Correct

Incorrect

**Figure 2.12** *Suturing a corneal laceration. A 10-0 nylon suture should be placed either full thickness or to the level of Descemet's membrane. The knot should be buried in the corneal stroma.*

lacerations may be oversewn in multiple directions (Fig. 2.14). If corneal tissue is missing, a purse-string suture technique using 10-0 nylon may be useful. The sutures are placed around the area of tissue loss and pulled tightly. This procedure may be augmented by using cyanoacrylate glue to ensure an aqueous tight closure. Cyanoacrylate glue is useful as a temporizing measure to treat corneal perforations and maintain the anterior chamber in patients with minor corneal tissue loss prior to penetrating keratoplasty.

## ASSOCIATED INJURIES

There is no universal agreement as to management of other intraocular injuries associated with corneal scleral lacerations. The author's team will remove a grossly ruptured lens that is obviously cataractous. Otherwise the laceration will be repaired and the patient re-evaluated after surgery. This allows for keratometry and biometry for intraocular lens calculation if cataract removal is necessary. Sometimes a lens that looks seriously compromised at the time of initial repair will maintain its clarity and not require removal.

If there is a combination of lacerated globe and eyelids (Fig. 2.15), the globe is repaired prior to the eyelids.

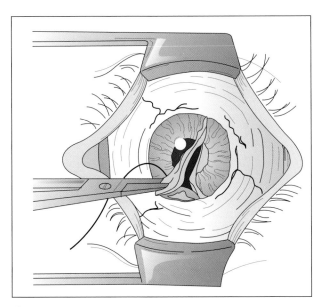

*a*

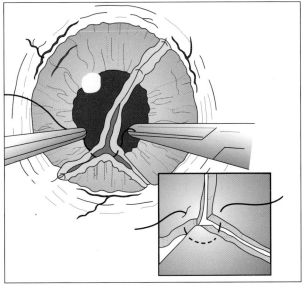

*b*

**Figure 2.13** *Stellate corneal laceration may be repaired using the halving technique as described for simple corneal lacerations. Suturing techniques need to be modified to close the stellate laceration effectively (b).*

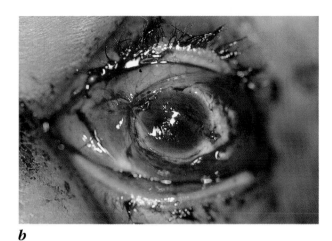

*a*

*b*

**Figure 2.14** *Successful repair of a large, complex, stellate corneal laceration (a) may tax the ingenuity of an experienced surgeon. An aqueous tight closure can usually be obtained, but may require innovative surgical techniques (Fig. 2.13) to close (b).*

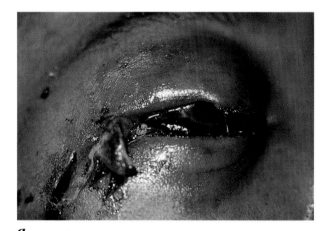

*a*

**Figure 2.15** *Knife wound to the lateral canthus (a) with accompanying occult posterior scleral laceration (b).*

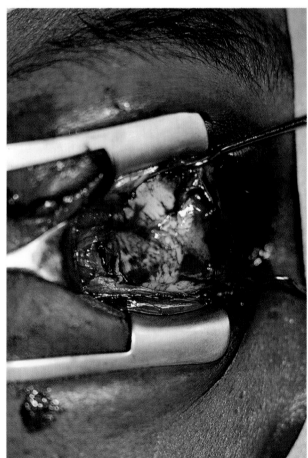

*b*

## BLUNT TRAUMA

An eye ruptured by blunt trauma (Fig. 2.2) has a much poorer prognosis than the eye lacerated by a sharp object. The rupture may be very obvious or occult. Ruptured globes occur in approximately

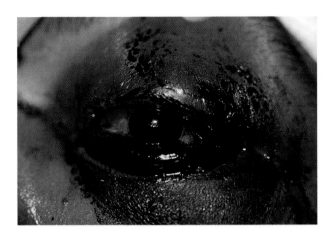

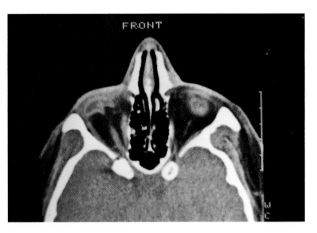

**Figure 2.16** *Subconjunctival hemorrhagic chemosis masking a scleral laceration.*

**Figure 2.17** *CT scan demonstrates obvious collapse of the globe.*

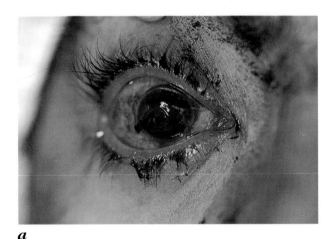

*a*

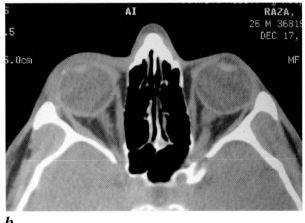

*b*

**Figure 2.18** *CT scan demonstrates collapse of the anterior chamber in an eye (a) with a corneal laceration. Note the foreign body evident in the anterior chamber (b).*

1.1–3.5% of patients suffering significant blunt ocular trauma. A scleral rupture may be obvious (Figs 2.2 and 2.6) or much more subtle. Extensive subconjunctival hemorrhage can obscure an anterior scleral rupture, while an intraocular hemorrhage can obscure a posterior scleral defect. Scleral ruptures invariably involve the underlying choroid or ciliary body. These structures are very vascular, hence hemorrhage often accompanies scleral ruptures. Extensive hyphema, subconjunctival or vitreous hemorrhage always accompanies a scleral rupture, but may occur in the absence of scleral rupture. Scleral ruptures occur in 25% of patients with traumatic hyphema and 22% of patients with exten-

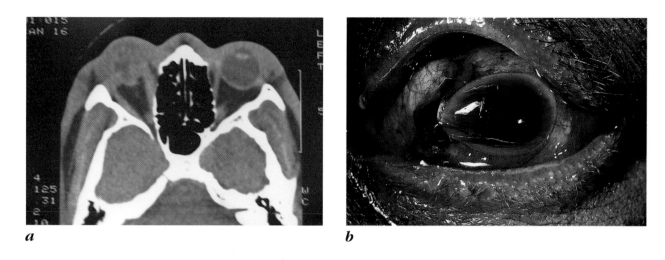

*a*                                          *b*

**Figure 2.19** *CT scan (a) demonstrates total disruption of a severely traumatized globe (b).*

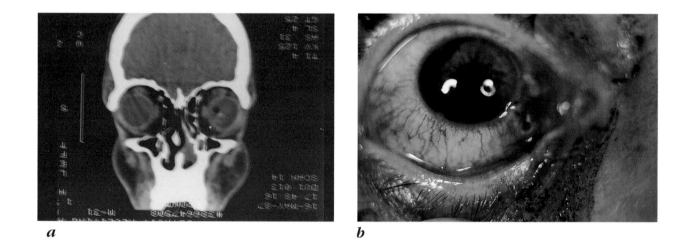

*a*                                          *b*

**Figure 2.20** *CT scan demonstrates intraocular birdshot (a) in a patient with an anterior segment wound (b).*

sive subconjunctival hemorrhagic chemosis (Fig. 2.16). What clinical findings should alert the clinician to the possibility of a scleral rupture in the patient presenting with blunt ocular trauma? Kylstra et al.[1] reviewed a series of patients with blunt ocular trauma. Twenty-nine patients had scleral ruptures,

and 273 patients did not. Patients with scleral ruptures tended to have the following characteristics: visual acuity of light perception (LP) or less; intraocular pressure of 5 mmHg or less; an abnormally deep or shallow anterior chamber; or media opacity preventing a view of the fundus with an indirect

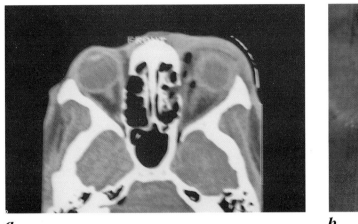
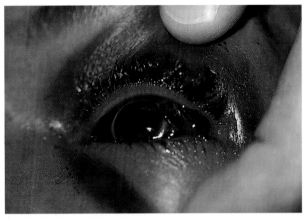

*a*  *b*

**Figure 2.21** *CT scan demonstrates intraorbital air and loss of normal ocular anatomy (a) in patient with pellet wound to eye (b).*

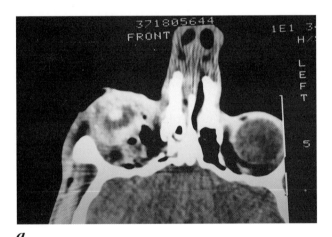
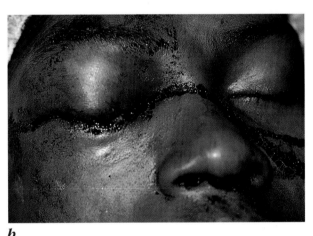

*a*  *b*

**Figure 2.22** *CT scan demonstrates marked disruption of eye (a) in patient with a gunshot wound to the eye and orbit (b). Swollen lids precluded a timely examination.*

ophthalmoscope. Other authors add an afferent pupillary defect and visual acuity of 20/400 or worse to the previous risk factors.[4] The present author also adds extensive conjunctival chemosis or hemorrhage to the indicators of predictive value. If there is reasonable suspicion that there is an occult rupture of the globe, it will be explored in the operating room. Considering the risks inherent in missing the diagnosis of a ruptured globe (endophthalmitis and sympathetic ophthalmia), not to mention the medicolegal ramifications, when in doubt these eyes should be explored. There is no stigma in a negative exploration of the globe. In one recent series, 68% of explorations were negative.[1]

## ROLE OF IMAGING STUDIES

Computed tomography is a valuable adjunct in evaluating patients with potential scleral ruptures. The posterior globe may appear obviously collapsed (Fig. 2.17) or deformed. The anterior chamber may be collapsed (Fig. 2.18); but here the diagnosis is usually obvious (Fig. 2.19). Computed tomography is most useful in evaluating eyes injured by a variety of pellet and gunshot wounds (Figs 2.20 and 2.21) or when the adnexal swelling is so great that it precludes a complete examination of the injured eye (Fig. 2.22). Computed tomography not only helps determine the integrity of the globe but also demonstrates the presence of intraocular foreign bodies and differentiates them from intraorbital foreign bodies.

## EXPLORING THE GLOBE

The same anesthetic precautions, preparation and draping procedures should be followed as with an obviously ruptured globe. A 360° conjunctival peritomy is performed. Relaxing incisions in each quadrant facilitate subsequent exposure. The insertions of the recti muscles are exposed and two adjacent muscles are gently isolated with muscle-hooks (Fig. 2.4). Gentle traction on each hook exposes the quadrant of the globe between the two muscles. This area is cleared with a cotton-tipped applicator; better exposure may be obtained by retracting the conjunctiva with a DesMarres retractor (Fig. 2.6). This procedure is repeated in each quadrant until the operator is comfortable that there is no scleral rupture present. An occult scleral rupture may be present under the insertion of a rectus muscle

(Fig. 2.7). If this is suspected, the muscle should be isolated, sutured and disinserted from the globe in such a manner that it can be reattached at the end of the procedure. Scleral ruptures when found should be sutured as described previously.

Double perforating injuries occur when a projectile penetrates the globe, traverses it, and exits at another site, usually posterior to the entry point. Management of these injuries is covered in the chapters on vitreo-retinal trauma and penetrating orbital injuries. The more posterior injury is usually self-sealing, difficult to access and may often be left unrepaired.

## SYMPATHETIC OPHTHALMIA

A study of trauma would not be complete without mentioning sympathetic ophthalmia (SO). SO is decidedly rare, with an incidence of approximately 0.1% of ocular perforations. Most ophthalmologists will practice their entire careers and never see a case. Their entire exposure to this entity is often studying for and taking the written and oral board examinations.

Sympathetic ophthalmia usually results from a perforating wound with incarcerated, prolapsed uvea. Microsurgical repair and compulsive removal of prolapsed uveal tissue from the wound has decreased the incidence of SO. Sympathetic ophthalmia is a panuveitis affecting the fellow, uninjured eye 2 weeks to 3 months after injury. Rarely, inflammation may develop in the fellow eye years after the injury has occurred. The injured eye is often also involved. Enucleation of the traumatized eye within 10 days of injury obviates the occurrence of SO. Once the disease occurs, enucleation of the injured eye has no effect on the outcome of the disease. Although rare, the potential development of sympathetic ophthalmia should be considered when deciding to enucleate a blind, injured eye. It should be remembered that enucleation within 14 days of injury protects the fellow eye from a potentially vision-threatening disease.

# REFERENCES

1    Kylstra J, Lamkin JC, Runyan DK. Clinical predictors of
     scleral rupture after blunt ocular trauma. *Am J Ophthalmol*
     1993; **115**: 530–5.

2    Werner MS, Dana M, Viana M, Shapiro M. Predictors of
     occult scleral rupture. *Ophthalmology* 1994; **101**: 1941–4.

3    Joseph E, Zak R, Smith S et al. Predictors of blinding or
     serious eye injury in blunt trauma. *J Trauma* 1992; **33**:
     19–23.

4    Esmaeli B, Elner S, Schork MA, Elner VM. Visual outcome
     and ocular survival after penetrating trauma. *Ophthalmology*
     1995; **102**: 393–400.

5    Barr CC. Prognostic factors in corneoscleral lacerations.
     *Arch Ophthalmol* 1983; **101**: 919–24.

6    Thompson JT, Parver LM, Enger C et al. Endophthalmitis
     after penetrating ocular injuries with retained intraocular
     foreign bodies. *Ophthalmology* 1993; **100**: 1468–74.

7    Thompson WS, Rubsamen PE, Flynn HW et al.
     Endophthalmitis following penetrating trauma.
     *Ophthalmology* 1995; **102**: 1696–701.

8    Ariyasu RG, Kumar S, La Bree LD et al. Microorganisms
     cultured from the anterior chamber of ruptured globes at
     the time of injury. *Am J Ophthalmol* 1995; **119**: 181–8.

# Chapter 3 Anterior segment injuries: blunt ocular trauma— What happens when the eye is struck by a blunt object?

The eye is surrounded and protected by the bony orbit. If a large object, for example, a tennis ball or a fist strikes the eye, most of its force is dissipated on the orbital rim. The lessened force upon the globe may cause expansion of the eye and orbital contents and fracture of the medial or inferior orbital walls (Fig. 3.1). A smaller object penetrating the orbital opening and striking the eye directly may cause a variety of ocular injuries ranging from minor to severe. Figure 3.2 demonstrates a blunt object, in this case, a golf ball, striking the eye directly. The cornea is pushed inwards compressing the fluid-filled globe. The globe expands circumferentially. At the moment of impact, a variety of injuries may occur, caused by compression and expansion of the globe.

If the trauma is sufficiently great, that is, the eye is struck directly by the golf ball, the globe may rupture. This usually occurs at its weakest points— the insertion of the recti muscles and the corneoscleral limbus (Fig. 3.3). Corneoscleral ruptures are obvious (Fig. 3.3). Lacerations at the insertions of the recti may be more difficult to detect (Fig. 3.4), especially if they are not suspected and sought.

The cornea rarely ruptures after blunt trauma unless it has been previously weakened by radial keratotomy or a pre-existent stromal thinning disorder. Blunt trauma may, however, cause significant loss of corneal endothelial cells compared with the contralateral uninjured eye. Cell loss probably results from the shock wave of the initial corneal trauma.

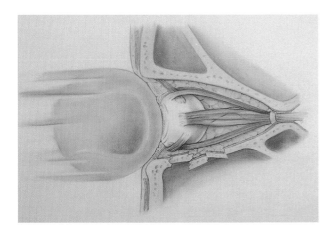

**Figure 3.1** *The eye is stuck by an object larger than the orbital opening, a tennis ball. Most of the force is dissipated on the orbital rim. Expansion of the eye and orbital contents may cause fractures of the medial wall and orbital floor. The eye is usually spared.*

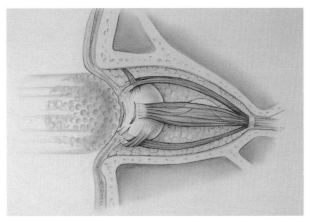

**Figure 3.2** *When the eye is struck by an object smaller than the orbital opening, here a golf ball, the force is directly applied to the eye, compressing the ocular contents, expanding the globe circumferentially and causing a variety of injuries.*

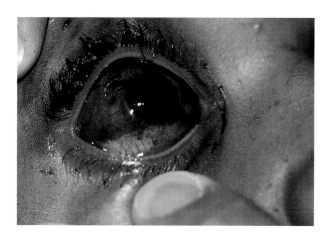

**Figure 3.3** *A ruptured globe occurring at the corneal scleral limbus.*

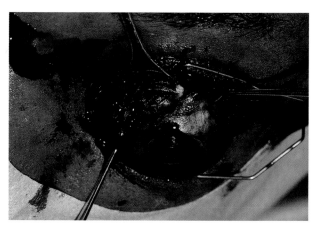

**Figure 3.4** *An occult globe rupture occurring at the insertion of the superior rectus muscle.*

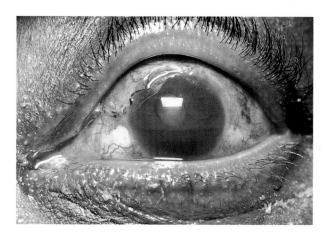

**Figure 3.5** *Traumatic hyphema: tearing of ciliary body blood vessels results in bleeding into the anterior chamber.*

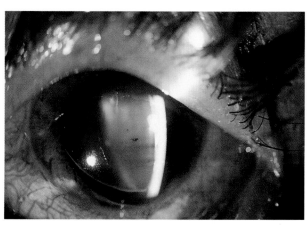

**Figure 3.6** *Subtle subluxation of the lens, evidenced by iridodonesis on slit-lamp examination.*

Recession of the anterior chamber angle indicates the presence of more extensive endothelial cell loss. Direct injury to the cornea may also cause tears in Descemet's membrane, as seen in patients with forceps injuries at birth.

The pupillary sphincter may rupture, causing radial tears and an irregular pupil. The iris may be avulsed from its attachment to the ciliary body (iridodialysis). This represents the area where the iris is thinnest and

most vulnerable to injury. The anterior chamber angle may be recessed, tearing ciliary body blood vessels and causing a traumatic hyphema (Fig. 3.5). Sequelae of angle recession may include early-onset and late-onset glaucoma due to interference with filtration. These glaucomas may also be the result of tears in the trabecular meshwork.

Cyclodialysis may occur, with the tear resulting in communication with the suprachoroidal space. These

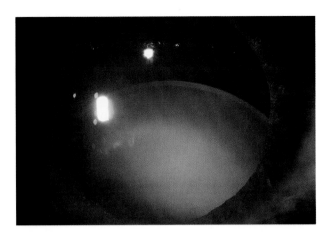

**Figure 3.7** *Obvious subluxation of the lens causing significant visual impairment.*

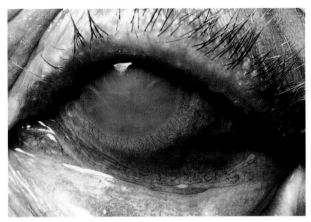

**Figure 3.8** *Subluxation of the lens into the anterior chamber with resultant corneal decompensation.*

patients may initially have markedly elevated intraocular pressure due to the concomitant hyphema and may later develop profound hypotony after the hyphema resolves.

Compression of the eye may also result in tears in the zonular ring suspending the crystalline lens. Mild zonular disruption may be evident by noting iridodonesis on careful slit-lamp examination. Dilated examination would then demonstrate subluxation of the lens (Fig. 3.6). More extensive zonular disruption may result in more obvious subluxation or dislocation of the lens (Fig. 3.7). The lens may be dislocated into the vitreous or into the anterior chamber (Fig. 3.8). Dislocation of the lens into the anterior chamber may result in a marked elevation of intraocular pressure and corneal decompensation. This represents a relative surgical emergency.

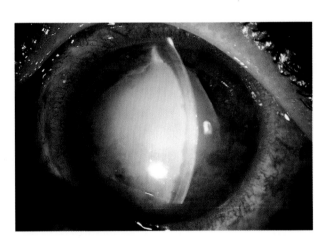

**Figure 3.9** *An obvious cataract rapidly develops after rupture of the anterior lens capsule.*

## SUBLUXATED LENSES

Depending on the degree of zonular disruption, the lens may be mildly subluxated (Fig. 3.6), significantly subluxated (Fig. 3.7), or dislocated into the anterior chamber or vitreous. Clear, mildly subluxated lenses (Fig.3.6) do not require treatment if vision is unimpaired. More severely subluxated lenses (Fig. 3.7) may or may not be removed. The patient in Fig. 3.7 had a significant subluxation of his lens in his only sighted eye. A visual acuity of 20/30 was

obtained with an aphakic contact lens, and no further treatment was offered.

An intact lens dislocated into the vitreous may be very well tolerated and make an interesting ophthalmoscopic finding for years, while causing little, if any, harm to the patient. If removal is necessary, it may be accomplished by vitreoretinal microsurgical techniques.

A lens dislocated into the anterior chamber (Fig. 3.8) is a relative surgical emergency. The cornea may

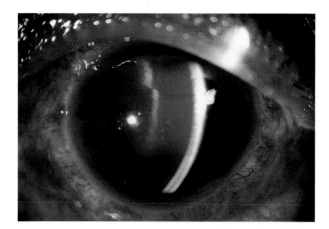

**Figure 3.10** *Traumatic hyphema with retrolenticular and vitreous hemorrhage secondary to disruption of the anterior hyaloid. This is a prerequisite for the development of ghost cell glaucoma.*

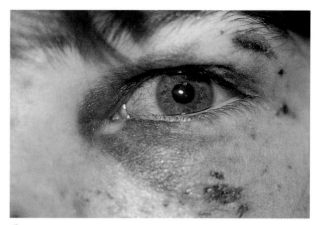

*a*

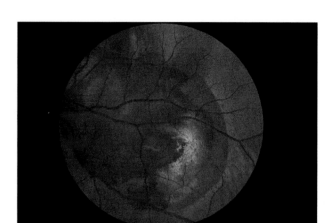

*b*

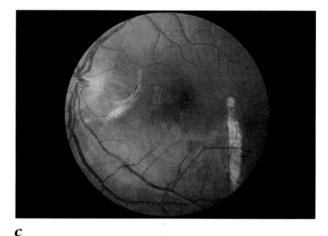

*c*

**Figure 3.11** *Boy struck in the left eye with a pool cue (a). Initial retinal hemorrhage obscures choroidal tears (b), which become obvious after blood has resorbed (c).*

rapidly decompensate due to damage to the endothelial cells. Pseudophakic patients may also have lenses dislocated after ocular trauma. This often results in rupture of the cataract wound and flattening of the anterior chamber. These lenses may be found in the fornix or in the disrupted wound. Subluxation of the pseudophakos into the anterior chamber requires emergent removal to avert further corneal endothelial damage and decompensation.

The anterior lens capsule may be disrupted by blunt injury, pushing the cornea and iris against it. A ring of pigment may be evident on the anterior lens capsule. This ring of Vossius is evidence for antecedent blunt ocular trauma. An anterior cataract may develop after such trauma. Rarely, the anterior lens capsule may be ruptured by blunt trauma and an obvious cataract may rapidly develop (Fig. 3.9).

Disruption of the eye at the ora serrata may result in retinal dialysis and detachment. Disruption of the hyaloid face may allow blood from the anterior chamber to enter the vitreous (Fig. 3.10); eventual reabsorption of the ghost cells and the macrophages ingesting them may clog the trabecular meshwork and cause ghost cell glaucoma.

Pressure and distention on the retina may cause choroidal tears. These may be hidden by overlying hemorrhage and be difficult to detect on initial examination. Their presence is obvious after the hemorrhage reabsorbs (Fig. 3.11). Depending upon their location, they may cause devastating visual loss.

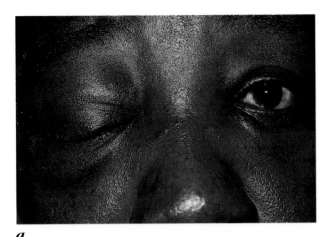

*a*

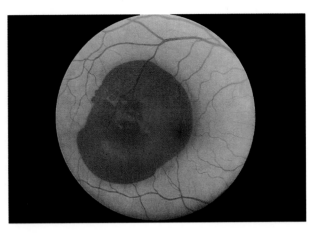

**Figure 3.13** *Large macular hemorrhage causes visual loss without a relative afferent pupillary defect.*

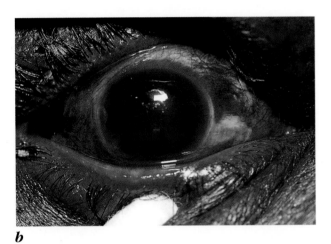

*b*

If vision is impaired and there is no obvious media opacity, for example, cataract, hyphema or vitreous hemorrhage, a traumatic optic neuropathy (see Chapter 11) should be considered or retinal hemorrhage or edema (see Chapter 5). Patients with traumatic injury to their optic nerves may have substantial visual loss and a totally normal examination except for the presence of an afferent pupillary defect. This should be sought and detected prior to dilatation in any patient with decreased vision after a periorbital injury. Patients with commotio retinae (Fig. 3.12) may also have significant visual loss; but there will be minimal, if any, afferent pupillary defect detectable in patients with maculopathies. Patients with macular hemorrhages (Fig. 3.13), may also have very significant visual loss; but no afferent pupillary defect.

## AIRBAG INJURIES

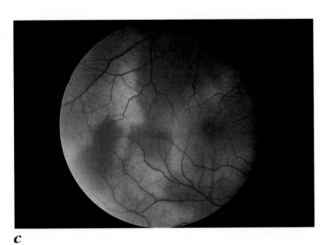

*c*

**Figure 3.12** *Patient with decreased vision after being struck in the right eye with a fist (a). Traumatic pupillary mydriasis (b) and clear ocular media. Extensive macular edema accounts for profound visual loss (c).*

Airbags prevent motor-vehicle-related injury and death. With the more extensive use of airbags, ocular injuries caused by inflation of the airbag are becoming more common. An airbag inflates at a velocity of 113–254 mph.[1] This imparts a great deal of kinetic energy to anything that it impacts. If it impacts the eye, classic sequelae of severe blunt ocular trauma

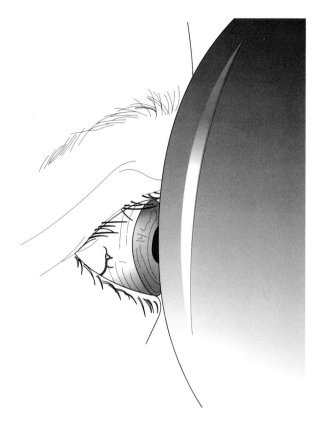

**Figure 3.14** *Airbag impacting face and cornea.*

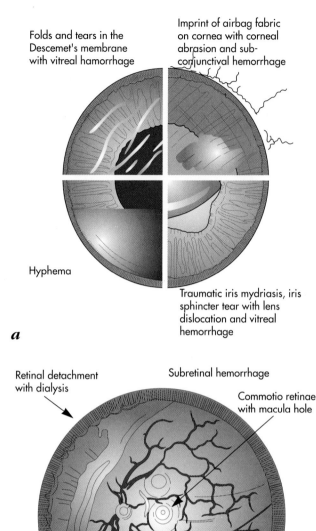

Folds and tears in the Descemet's membrane with vitreal hamorrhage

Imprint of airbag fabric on cornea with corneal abrasion and sub-conjunctival hemorrhage

Hyphema

Traumatic iris mydriasis, iris sphincter tear with lens dislocation and vitreal hemorrhage

*a*

Retinal detachment with dialysis

Subretinal hemorrhage

Commotio retinae with macula hole

Choroidal ruptures

Retinal detachment with tear

*b*

**Figure 3.15** *Diagrammatic representation of potential sequelae of airbag injuries to the eye.*

may result (Figs 3.14 and 3.15). If a potentially sharp object lies between the driver's face and the expanding airbag, corneoscleral lacerations have been reported. The patient in Fig. 3.16 was a Pakistani-trained medical resident involved in an automobile collision. His airbags expanded, sparing him significant bodily injury; however his glasses were not made of safety glass or plastic; they shattered, and the shards of glass lacerated his cornea (Fig. 3.17). The concussive force of airbag impact has been reported to cause corneoscleral laceration in the absence of sharp, hard objects.[2] Wearing safety glasses while driving a car with airbags might be prudent until an airbag is designed that minimizes the risk of ocular injury.

## TRAUMATIC HYPHEMA

There is no universal agreement as to the proper management of patients with traumatic hyphema.

The literature is obfuscated by many, often poorly controlled, studies comparing various treatment regimens with one another and with the author's or institution's previous experience. There are vocative

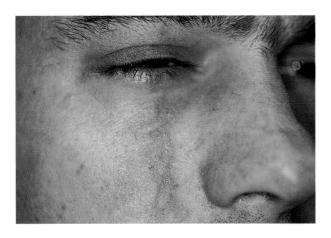

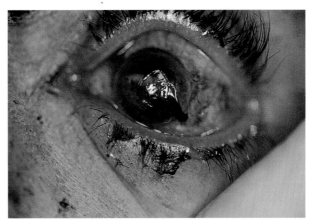

**Figure 3.16** *Patient struck by airbag. Note the telltale markings on the face and periorbital region.*

**Figure 3.17** *Corneal laceration resulting from shattered glasses.*

arguments for and against bed rest versus ambulation; unilateral or bilateral patching; outpatient versus inpatient treatment; systemic steroids versus no steroids; whether or not to use antifibrinolytics; total cycloplegia versus partial cycloplegia versus miosis; and the list goes on. A recent survey of ophthalmologists in the UK found little agreement on whether bed rest, patching or topical medications were indicated but almost universal agreement that systemic steroids and antifibrinolytics are not indicated.[3] There is little argument, however, that successful treatment of traumatic hyphema entails identifying risk factors for rebleeding, proper medical management of intraocular pressure elevation and ocular inflammation, and prompt surgical management when medical management fails.[4] Appropriate medical treatment is predicated upon the patient involved. Populations with high incidences of rebleeding after traumatic hyphema, for example, inner-city black people, probably benefit from medications that decrease the incidence of rebleeding,[5] while patients with a low incidence of rebleeding, for example, northern European Caucasians, do not require as aggressive medical management.[6,7] These patients rarely rebleed, and treatment with antifibrinolytics has rarely been shown to be more beneficial in preventing rebleeding than in the untreated group. Patients with sickle cell trait have potentially more complications from traumatic hyphema and need to be treated more aggressively.

Amicar (epsilon-amino caproic acid) given orally at 100 mg/kg every 4 hours for 5 days (not to exceed 30 g/day) has been shown in double-blind controlled studies to decrease the incidence of secondary hemorrhage in patients at high risk for secondary hemorrhage.[8] Amicar treatment, however, prolongs the time it takes blood to reabsorb from the anterior chamber; and in patients at low risk for rebleeding, it is of little benefit.[9]

Another antifibrinolytic agent, transexamic acid, 25 mg/kg every 8 hours (not to exceed 1500 mg every 8 hours) given orally, has been shown to decrease the incidence of rebleeding from 10% to 3% with no significant ocular or systemic side-effects.[10]

Antifibrinolytic agents should be used in patients at high risk for secondary hemorrhage from traumatic hyphema.[5,8] Since, usually, only patients who rebled require surgery, the use of antifibrinolytic agents should be weighed against the risks of rebleeding, general anesthesia and surgery.[11]

Practical and appropriate management of traumatic hyphema depends on the patient involved and the physician's comfort level with the patient's compliance. The basic tenets of management include a careful examination to rule out an occult ruptured globe and consideration of retinal or optic nerve injury that may be obscured by the blood in the anterior chamber. Injuries to the macula occur at the time of the initial trauma, and there is little to be done for them acutely. After concurrent injuries have

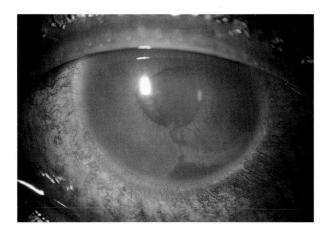

**Figure 3.18** *Small, uncomplicated hyphema.*

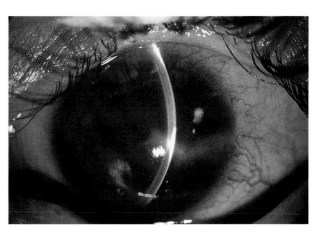

**Figure 3.19** *Total (eight-ball) hyphema.*

been rule out, management consists of bed rest to minimize secondary hemorrhage and daily examinations to detect and treat elevated intraocular pressure. In some patients, this may require hospitalization, strict bed rest and sedation.[5] Other patients may be adequately treated in a quiet home environment.[7,9] There can be no hard and fast rules; this decision must be made by the treating physician's evaluation of the individual patient's needs and abilities. One would be much more inclined to send a patient home to a quiet environment with an intelligent, reliable family member than to send a child home to a household containing many other siblings living in an uncontrolled, undisciplined environment. Restricting activity is necessary to prevent or at least minimize the risk of secondary hemorrhage. Daily examination is necessary to detect and treat elevated intraocular pressure with or without secondary hemorrhage. Are daily visits to the doctor's office more activity than the patient should have to minimize the risk of secondary hemorrhage? The author thinks so, and his own prejudice is to hospitalize these patients and treat them as little as possible. The eye is patched and the patch removed only to examine the patient on a daily basis or to instill medications.

An uncomplicated hyphema (Fig. 3.18) usually resorbs within 3–5 days, and the risk of rebleeding is decreased. These patients may slowly return to a more active lifestyle, although full activity is limited until they have undergone their complete eye examination three weeks after injury. At this time, gonioscopy is performed to document angle recession and a complete retinal examination with scleral depression is performed to detect any asymptomatic retinal holes or tears.

## SURGICAL MANAGEMENT

Patients who rebleed either after initial evaluation or before their initial examination are those patients with a complicated clinical course that may require surgical intervention. A total (eight-ball) hyphema (Fig. 3.19) or a hyphema that has rebled (Fig. 3.20) may cause visual dysfunction by blood-staining of the corneal endothelium (Fig. 3.21) or elevated intraocular pressure from blockage of the trabecular meshwork.

Corneal endothelial blood-staining (Fig. 3.21) classically begins after 5 days of elevated intraocular pressure. In reality it may occur much more rapidly if the intraocular pressure is markedly elevated. Endothelial blood-staining will eventually resolve after normalization of intraocular pressure.

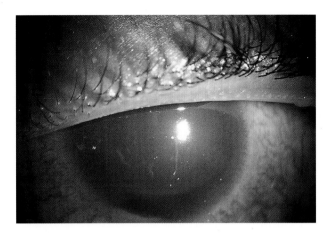

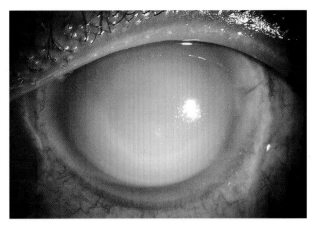

**Figure 3.20** *Rebleeding into the anterior chamber causing a secondary hyphema.*

**Figure 3.21** *Extensive corneal blood-staining.*

Elevated intraocular pressure is the potentially blinding and treatable complication of traumatic hyphema. Elevated intraocular pressure should be aggressively lowered medically or surgically. Topical beta-blockers and iopamidol combined with systemic acetazolamide and hyperosmotic agents are the mainstays of medical management. These medications lower intraocular pressure; but sustaining the lowered pressure may be difficult. This is the role of surgery.

Classically, hyphema surgery has entailed irrigating and aspirating the blood from the anterior chamber. More recently, anterior chamber irrigation and aspiration has been combined with trabeculectomy and peripheral iridectomy to maintain a lower intraocular pressure while the residual blood resorbs and the trabecular meshwork function normalizes.[12] If the intraocular pressure is sufficiently elevated to require evacuation of the hyphema, the trabecular meshwork is probably dysfunctional enough to require trabeculectomy to maintain control of the intraocular pressure. For the experienced surgeon, this is the procedure of choice.

To reiterate, successful treatment of traumatic hyphema entails identification of risk factors, appropriate medical therapy and prompt surgical intervention when medical management fails. The author's experience is that hyphemas are either very easy to manage, with the blood reabsorbing spontaneously in 3–5 days (Figs 3.5 and 3.18) or very difficult, with multiple episodes of secondary hemorrhage and marked elevation of intraocular pressure that is often refractory to medical management (Figs 3.19 and 3.20). These patients should be operated upon as soon as it is evident that their intraocular pressure cannot be controlled.

## REFERENCES

1 Kuhn M, Morris R, Witherspoon CD et al. Air bag: friend or foe? *Arch Ophthalmol* 1993; **111**: 1333–4.

2 Baker R, Flowers CW, Singh P et al. Corneoscleral laceration caused by airbag trauma. *Am J Ophthalmol* 1996; **121**: 709–11.

3 Little BC, Aylward GW. The medical management of traumatic hyphema. *J R Soc Med* 1993; **86**: 458–9.

4 Gottsch JD. Hyphema—diagnosis and management. *Retina* 1990; **10 (suppl 1)**: 565–71.

5 Spoor TC, Kwitko GM, O'Grady JA, Ramocki JM. Traumatic hyphema in an urban population. *Am J Ophthalmol* 1990; **109**: 23–7.

6 Volpe NJ, Larrison WI, Hersh PS et al. Secondary hyphema in traumatic hyphema. *Am J Ophthalmol* 1991; **112**: 507–13.

7 Agapitos PJ, Nael LT, Clarke WM. Traumatic hyphema in children. *Ophthalmology* 1987; **94**: 1238–41.

8 Kutner B, Fourman S, Brien K et al. Aminocaproic acid reduces risk of secondary hemorrhage in patients with traumatic hyphema. *Arch Ophthalmol* 1987; **105**: 206–8.

9 Kraft SP, Christianson JD, Crawford JS. Traumatic hyphema in children. Treatment with ACA. *Ophthalmology* 1987; **94**: 1232–7.

10 Deans R, Noel LP, Clarke WM. Oral administration of transexamic acid in management of traumatic hyphema. *Can J Ophthalmol* 1992; **27**: 181–3.

11 Thomas MA, Parrish RK, Feuer WJ. Rebleeding after traumatic hyphema. *Am J Ophthalmol* 1986; **104**: 206–10.

12 Graul TA, Ruttum MS, Lloyd MA et al. Trabeculectomy for traumatic hyphema. *Am J Ophthalmol* 1994; **117**: 155–9.

# Chapter 4 Thermal and caustic ocular trauma

Chemical and thermal injuries to the eye vary greatly in both severity and prognosis. A mild injury, de-epithelializing the cornea (Fig. 4.1), may be very painful but, if infection is prevented, will heal completely with no loss of visual function. Severe alkali burns (Fig. 4.2) have a very poor visual prognosis in spite of often heroic treatment. The visual outcome correlates with the severity of the injury at presentation.[1] There is no good treatment for severe alkali burns. Alkalis, and some very strong acids, penetrate tissue rapidly, saponify cell membranes, denature collagen, cause vascular thrombosis and rapidly destroy the eye and useful vision (Fig. 4.2).[2] On the contrary, weak acids do not penetrate tissue well. They precipitate protein on contact, protecting the underlying corneal stroma and anterior segment. Most thermal injuries behave in a similar fashion. The epithelial cell protein is precipitated, resulting in a ground glass appearance of the cornea that peels away revealing clear corneal stroma (Figs 4.1 and 4.3).

The severity of a chemical burn to the eye is related to the concentration, volume and duration of contact of the chemical with the eye. Very concentrated acids and alkalis are more toxic than dilute solutions. The sooner a caustic substance is removed or irrigated from the eye the better. Strong alkalis penetrate the anterior chamber almost immediately and continue to penetrate until the solution is neutralized in the external eye. Hence the importance of immediate irrigation and removal of particulate matter. The eye should be irrigated with any nontoxic solution that is available. Continued irrigation may be more comfortable with Balance salt solution (Allergan, Irvine, CA)[3] but is equally effective with lactated Ringer's or normal saline. Do not wait for a sterile, 'correct' irrigating solution. Irrigate the eye with whatever nontoxic solution is available (water) and switch to a more comfortable solution when it is available. Particulate matter (plaster, lime powder, lye with molasses) should be swabbed from the cul-de-sac with a Q-tip while irrigating the eye. The upper

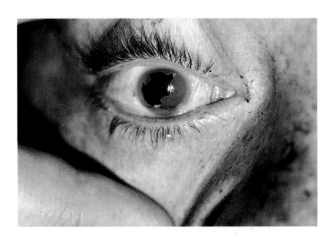

**Figure 4.1** *Thermal injury to the cornea causing an isolated epithelial defect. Complete recovery is expected.*

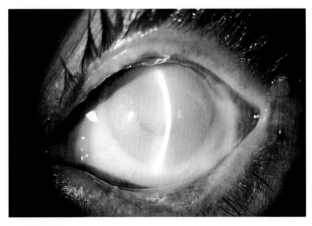

**Figure 4.2** *Severe (grade 4) alkali injury to the eye. Note near total opacification of the cornea. Iris details are not evident. This burn has a dismal prognosis.*

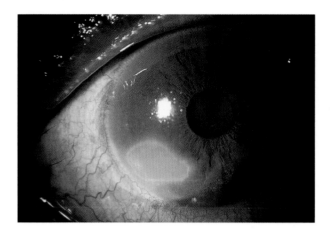

**Figure 4.3** *Acid burn to cornea causing a localized epithelial defect.*

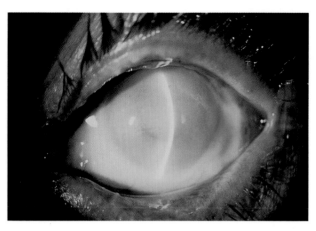

**Figure 4.4** *Severe ocular alkali burn. Note opacification of the cornea and blanching of the limbus.*

eyelid should be double-everted to detect occult particulate matter in the upper fornix. Irrigation should continue for 30–60 minutes until the pH of the external eye is neutralized. To reiterate, the most beneficial treatment for ocular alkali burns is immediate, copious irrigation with a nontoxic fluid and removal of particulate matter from the eye.[4] In a large series of chemical burns, 56% of workplace injuries and 42% of home injuries received the benefit of immediate irrigation. Those patients receiving immediate irrigation had less ocular damage, fewer surgical procedures, less time in the hospital, and a better visual prognosis.[5] This study underlines the importance of immediate irrigation with whatever nontoxic liquid is available.

What happens when a strong alkali enters the eye? The patient has extreme pain due to stimulation of free sensory nerve endings in the skin, conjunctiva and cornea. The pain is exacerbated by a rapid rise in intraocular pressure caused by shrinkage of collagen in the outer coats of the eye, followed by release of intraocular prostaglandins. The corneal stroma opacifies, and the exposed conjunctiva whitens as the alkali rapidly passes through them (Fig. 4.4).

As the solution permeates the anterior chamber, the pH rises, cells lyse, the blood–aqueous barrier breaks down, and a fibrinous exudate may fill the anterior chamber. The elevated pH is not compatible with normal cellular function and the iris, ciliary body, trabecular meshwork and lens may be damaged. Any combination of glaucoma, hypotony, mydriasis and

cataract may follow. Extensive damage to the ciliary body may cause profound hypotony and phthisis bulbi. Damage to the trabecular meshwork may cause markedly elevated intraocular pressure. These changes are rarely compatible with restoration of useful vision. This is why there is a plethora of older literature advocating anterior chamber paracentesis and instillation of a Tris buffer or balanced salt solution into the anterior chamber as soon after an alkali burn as feasible.[2] In reality it probably makes little difference to the ultimate outcome.

Repair of the corneal epithelium is a potential problem. If only the corneal epithelium is involved (Figs 4.1 and 4.3) the defect will be repaired like a simple abrasion by migration of epithelial cells. If there is significant damage to the adjacent conjunctiva (Figs 4.2 and 4.4), epithelial migration may be delayed for several weeks. The persistent epithelial defects may result in corneal ulceration or perforation. Some authors advocate immediate conjunctival recession with either mucous membrane grafting or, more recently, conjunctival transplantation.[6] Removal of the injured conjunctiva reduces exposure of the corneal stroma to collagenases and decreases the risk of corneal melting. Other goals of conjunctival recession and transplantation are stabilization of tear film, decrease in vascularization and epithelial erosions. More recently, others have described early debridement of necrotic tissue from the conjunctiva and sclera accompanied by a rotational flap of Tenon's capsule from the equatorial region of the eye,

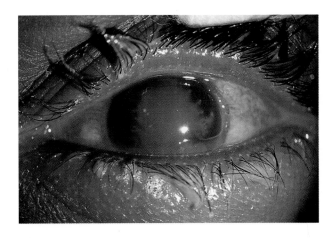

**Figure 4.5** *Grade 1 ocular burn involving only the loss of corneal epithelium.*

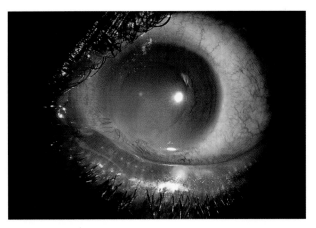

**Figure 4.6** *Grade 2 ocular burn demonstrates stromal haze and a small amount of limbal ischemia (less than one-third).*

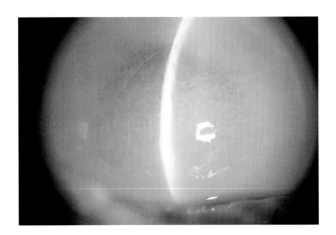

**Figure 4.7** *Grade 3 ocular burn manifests widespread stromal haze and significant (one-third to a half) stromal haze.*

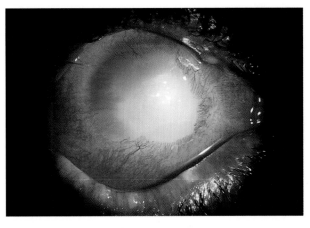

**Figure 4.8** *Grade 4 ocular burn. The cornea is opaque, the iris and pupil cannot be visualized, and there is extensive limbal ischemia (more than half).*

keeping the blood supply intact.[7] These eyes are then treated with high doses of topical corticosteroids to suppress reactive inflammation and prevent corneal neovascularization. The goals of this procedure are healing of the ulcerated and necrotic sclera and allowing rapid regeneration of conjunctival and corneal epithelium. More recently, Reim has advocated adding artificial epithelium to the tenonplasty.[8] Others have suggested conjunctival and stem cell allografts to re-epithelialize the corneal surface.[9] These techniques may be worth trying since there is still no good treatment or combination of treatments for severe ocular alkali burns.

For prognostication, ocular burns may be graded on a continuum of severity.[10] A grade 1 ocular burn (Fig. 4.5) only involves corneal epithelial loss. There is no ischemia of the conjunctival vessels, and the prognosis for visual function is excellent. A grade 2

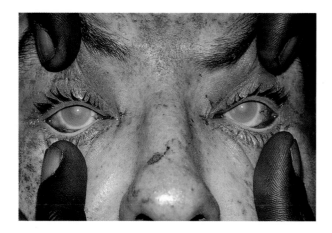

**Figure 4.9** *Bilateral grade 4 alkali burns caused by sodium hydroxide.*

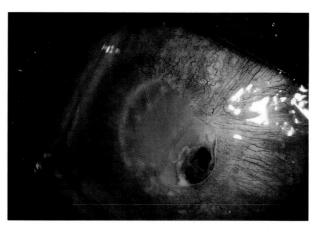

**Figure 4.10** *Limbal necrosis and a failed corneal graft after attempt to maintain integrity of the globe in grade 4 corneal burn (Fig. 4.8).*

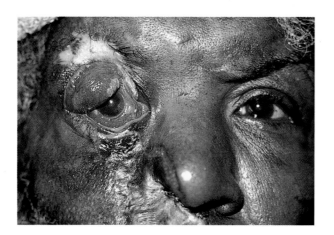

**Figure 4.11** *Severe burn to the eyelids sparing the underlying eye.*

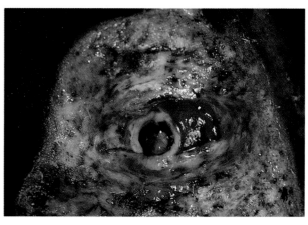

**Figure 4.12** *Severe burn to the eyelid with total destruction of the underlying eye.*

burn demonstrates epithelial loss with some stromal haze (Fig. 4.6). Less than one-third of the limbus is ischemic and visual prognosis is good; however, due to the corneal stromal involvement some scarring will persist. A grade 3 ocular burn manifests widespread stromal haze with obscuration of iris details (Fig. 4.7). Ischemia is evident from one-third to half of the limbus. With a grade 4 ocular burn, the cornea is opaque, there is no view of iris or pupil, and more than half of the limbus is ischemic (Fig. 4.8). Grade 3 and 4 burns have a dismal prognosis for recovery of visual function (Fig. 4.9). Eyes with severe alkali burns are prone to corneal melting and scleral necrosis. Emergent corneal grafting in an effort to maintain the integrity of the globe is often doomed to further melting and necrosis (Fig. 4.10).

Visual prognosis from ocular burns is also dependent upon concomitant damage to the eyelids and

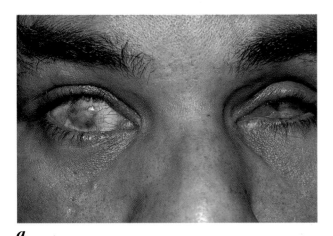

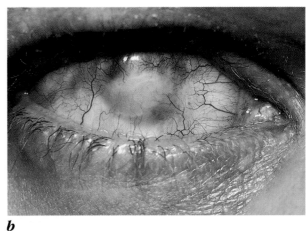

*a*                                           *b*

**Figure 4.13** *Late appearance of a severe ocular alkali injury. The left eye has been eviscerated. The right eye has no useful visual function. The cornea is opacified and neovascularization is evident (b).*

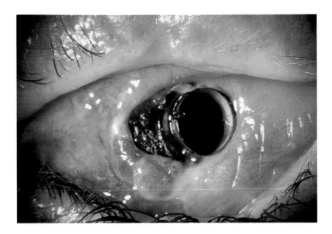

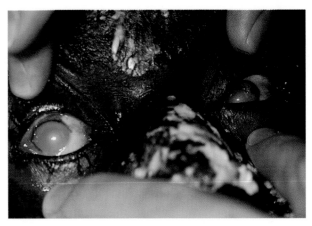

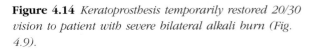

**Figure 4.14** *Keratoprosthesis temporarily restored 20/30 vision to patient with severe bilateral alkali burn (Fig. 4.9).*

**Figure 4.15** *Alkali burn to both eyes after assault with sodium hydroxide.*

conjunctiva. As mentioned in Chapter 6, the eye is often spared with thermal injuries to the eyelids (Fig. 4.11). More severe burns may cause injury to the underlying eye. This is often the result of a burn inflicted upon an unconscious individual (Fig. 4.12). Both patients in Figs 4.10 and 4.11 were intoxicated and fell asleep against a radiator. The patient in Fig. 4.10 had a blood alcohol level of 0.3 mg/ml, was aroused by the pain, and spared his eye. The patient

in Fig. 4.11 had a blood alcohol in excess of 0.5 mg/ml and did not awaken. The burn destroyed both the eyelids and the underlying eye.

The visual prognosis for severe ocular burns is dismal. The patient in Fig. 4.13 lost his left eye to an alkali burn and has severe injury to the right eye precluding useful visual function. Multiple penetrating keratoplasties with or without immunosuppression (cyclosporin A) and prosthetic corneas (Fig.

4.14) often fail to restore visual function for any length of time.[5] The absolute best treatment for ocular burns is prevention. Industry has made great progress in protecting workers from on-the-job ocular burns. Rules mandating protective eyewear are an excellent start, but they must be enforced by regulation and education of the workers. In a survey of eye injuries in the chemical industry in Great Britain, the incidence of eye injuries was 11.4/1000 workers per year. Forty-five percent of these injuries were caused by chemicals. Thirty-three percent of the injured workers were not wearing the mandated eye protection at the time of injury. The incidence of industrial eye injuries may be lowered by protection, legislation and education.[11]

Education is the key issue. One cannot legislate how people behave in their own homes, and a significant number of ocular burns occur in the home environment. In one series,[1] 37% of ocular burns occurred at home as opposed to 60% at work. The remainder may result from assaults and are often the most devastating (Fig. 4.15). These injuries often occur in large inner city areas, inflicted by a paramour using household lye (sodium hydroxide). The victim is often abruptly interrupted, turns and faces his attacker. His wide open eyes are very susceptible to the ensuing chemical injury as the solution is thrown in the victim's face. The ensuing visual results and complications are devastating. These victims are usually of low income, living in high-density housing, with a history of alcoholism, drug abuse and prior assaults.[2]

It is important to educate patients as to the potential dangers and devastation caused by caustic ocular injuries. Care in handling potentially caustic material and the wearing of safety glasses when dealing with potentially dangerous situations will help decrease the incidence of these visually devastating injuries.

## REFERENCES

1  Kulkelkorn R, Luft J, Kottek AA et al. Chemical and thermal eye burns in the residential area of Aachen. *Klin Monatsbl Augenheilkd* 1993; **202**: 34–42.

2  Pfister R. Chemical injuries of the eye. *Ophthalmology* 1983; **90**: 1246–53.

3  Herr RD, White GL, Bernhisul K et al. Clinical comparison of ocular irrigation fluids following chemical injuries. *Am J Emerg Med* 1991; **9**: 228–31.

4  Gangadhar DV, Kenyon KR, Wagoner IA. The surgical management of chemical ocular injuries. *Int Ophthalmol Clin* 1995; **35**: 63–9.

5  Kulkelkorn R, Kottek A, Schrag N, Reim M. Poor prognosis of severe chemical and thermal eye burns: the need for adequate emergency care and adequate prevention. *Arch Occup Environ Health* 1995; **67**: 281–4.

6  Thoft RA. Indications for conjunctival transplantation. *Ophthalmology* 1982; **89**: 335–40.

7  Teping C, Reim M. Tenonplasty as a new surgical treatment for severe chemical eye burns. *Klin Monatsbl Augenheilkd* 1989; **194**: 1–5.

8  Reim M. A new treatment concept for severe caustic and thermal lesions of the eye. *Klin Monatsbl Augenheilkd* 1990; **196**: 1–5.

9  Coster DJ, Aggarwal RK, Williams KA. Surgical management of ocular surface disorders using conjunctival and stem cell allografts. *Br J Ophthalmol* 1995; **79**: 977–82.

10  Eagling EM, Roper-Hall MJ. *Eye Injuries*. (Philadelphia: JB Lippincott, 1986): 4.6–4.7.

11  Griffeth GA, Jones MP. Eye injury and eye protection: a survey of the chemical industry. *Occup Med (Eng)* 1994; **44**: 37–40.

# Chapter 5 Posterior segment trauma

*Dean Eliott*

## NONPENETRATING POSTERIOR SEGMENT TRAUMA

A nonpenetrating injury results from blunt trauma to the eye with the globe remaining intact. Posterior segment manifestations include commotio retinae, choroidal rupture, sclopetaria, macular holes, and conditions associated with traumatic retinal detachment such as vitreous base avulsion, retinal dialysis, retinal tears, and giant retinal tears.

Mechanisms of posterior segment involvement from blunt trauma include coup injury, contrecoup injury, and direct ocular compression. A coup injury is damage at the site of impact, as seen with sclopetaria. In a contrecoup injury, damage occurs at tissue interfaces opposite the site of impact. This occurs with commotio retinae, posterior choroidal rupture, and traumatic macular holes. Anteroposterior ocular compression results in equatorial stretching because the eye has a fixed volume, and vitreous base avulsion and retinal dialysis occur via that mechanism.[1,2]

## COMMOTIO RETINAE

In 1873, Berlin described retinal whitening following blunt trauma to the globe, and the condition became known as Berlin's edema. Now known as commotio retinae, this relatively common condition is characterized by transient opacification of the deep retina opposite the site of impact (a contrecoup injury). The findings may vary from a small area of subtle retinal opacification (Fig. 5.1) to widespread marked retinal whitening (Fig. 5.2). If the posterior pole is involved, the fovea is often spared, resulting in a pseudo-cherry-red spot (Fig. 5.3). Commotio retinae has been documented several hours following an injury, and it usually progressively resolves within hours or days.

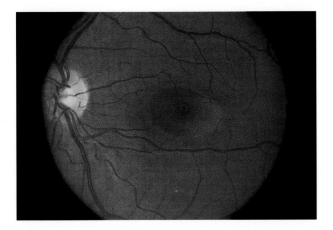

**Figure 5.1** *Commotio retinae: subtle retinal whitening temporal to fovea after blunt trauma.*

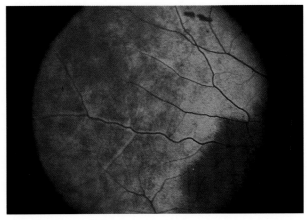

**Figure 5.2** *Commotio retinae: marked peripheral retinal whitening and small intraretinal hemorrhages following blunt trauma.*

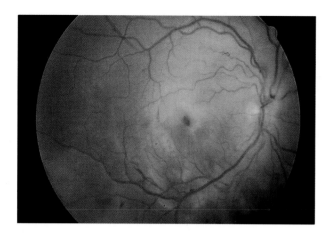

**Figure 5.3** *Commotio retinae: posterior deep retinal whitening demonstrating a pseudo-cherry-red spot.*

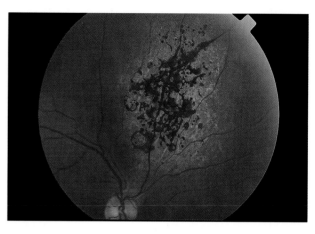

**Figure 5.4** *Intraretinal perivascular bone spicule pigmentation following commotio retinae.*

Rarely, mottling of the retinal pigment epithelium or intraretinal pigment deposition results (Fig. 5.4). When commotio retinae develops in the macula, vision may be decreased. Visual acuity usually returns to normal when the whitening resolves; however, in severe cases, visual loss may be permanent.[3]

The pathogenesis of commotio retinae is based on angiographic and histopathologic studies. The blood–retinal barrier appears to be intact, as demonstrated by numerous angiographic studies in both animals and humans with commotio retinae.[4–6] Histopathologic studies indicate disruption of photoreceptor outer segments[5,7] and the susceptibility of the outer segments may be attributed to the architecture of the retinal Müller cells. Müller cells occupy the retina from the internal limiting membrane to the photoreceptor inner segment and support all cellular layers except the photoreceptor outer segments.

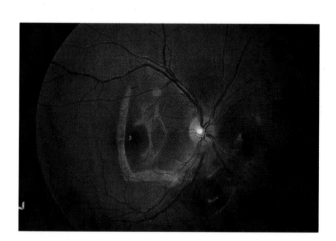

**Figure 5.5** *Typical crescent-shaped choroidal rupture oriented concentric with the disc margin.*

## CHOROIDAL RUPTURE

Indirect choroidal ruptures are crescent-shaped lesions of the posterior pole concentric with the disc margin (Fig. 5.5). They are located opposite the site of impact (a contrecoup injury) and are actually tears of the choroid, Bruch's membrane, and retinal pigment epithelium. Initially a subretinal hemor-

rhage is often present due to injury to the choriocapillaris, and the curvilinear lesion may not be visible until the overlying hemorrhage resorbs. Fluorescein angiography may help detect choroidal ruptures beneath a subretinal hemorrhage (Fig. 5.6). Visual acuity is affected when the rupture or the

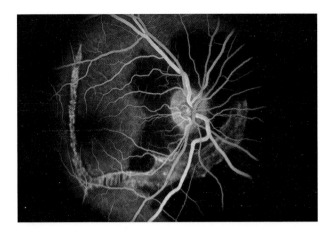

**Figure 5.6** *Same patient as in Fig. 5.5. Fluorescein angiography demonstrates curvilinear choroidal rupture. Although thin subretinal peripapillary hemorrhage blocks the underlying choroidal fluorescence, the full extent of the choroidal rupture is visible.*

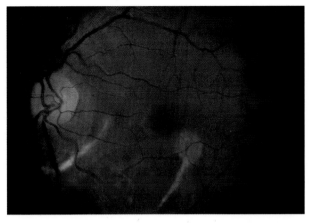

**Figure 5.8** *Same patient as in Fig. 5.7 with subretinal fluid associated with choroidal neovascularization.*

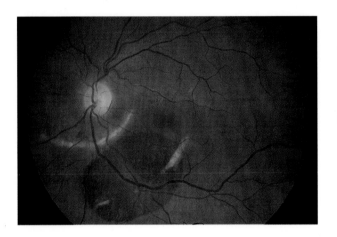

**Figure 5.7** *Two crescent-shaped choroidal ruptures; one is partially obscured by subretinal hemorrhage.*

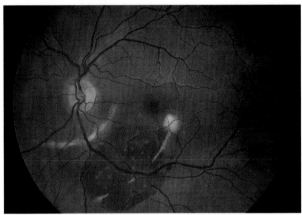

**Figure 5.9** *Same patient as in Fig. 5.8 following photocoagulation.*

accompanying subretinal hemorrhage involves the macula. With time, hyperpigmentation may develop at the margins of the healed lesions.[8] The most important potential sequela is choroidal neovascularization from the margins, which may develop at any time and may cause significant visual loss. Any visual changes should prompt an immediate evaluation. If subretinal fluid, hemorrhage, or lipid are present, fluorescein angiography is indicated to rule out choroidal neovascularization, and photocoagulation may be beneficial in these patients (Figs 5.7–5.9).[9] Histopathologic reports[8] indicate that new

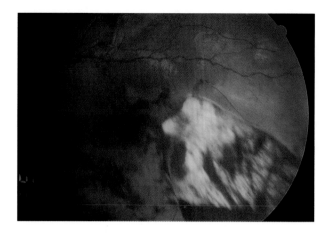

**Figure 5.10** *Sclopetaria: inferotemporal area of the bare sclera.*

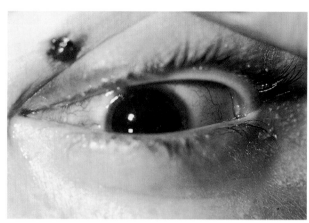

**Figure 5.11** *Left upper lid penetration site from BB pellet.*

choroidal blood vessels are common in the healing process and that these vessels often spontaneously regress.

## SCLOPETARIA

Sclopetaria occurs when a high-velocity projectile, typically a shotgun or BB pellet, strikes or passes tangential to the globe. This rare condition, also known as chorioretinal rupture, is characterized by rupture of the retina, retinal pigment epithelium, Bruch's membrane, and choroid. These tissues retract as a single unit, revealing the underlying sclera which becomes visible ophthalmoscopically (Fig. 5.10).[9] During the acute injury, however, overlying vitreous hemorrhage and adjacent intraretinal and subretinal hemorrhage may obscure these findings (Figs 5.11 and 5.12). The risk of acute retinal detachment is low, but long-term follow-up is essential. Late complications include retinal detachment and vitreous hemorrhage.[9]

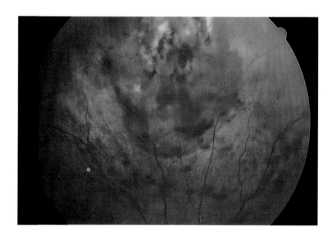

**Figure 5.12** *Sclopetaria: superior fundus of patient in Fig. 5.11.*

## TRAUMATIC MACULAR HOLE

Macular holes may be caused by a variety of conditions, and the clinical features are similar regardless of the cause. After blunt trauma, 6% of eyes develop a macular hole.[10] The vitreous is firmly adherent to the retina at the fovea, and a sudden traumatic separation of the posterior hyaloid from the retina may result in a dehiscence of retinal tissue at the fovea.[11] Alternatively, macular hole formation may occur slowly, resulting from trauma-induced cystoid macular edema, cyst coalescence, and eventual rupture of both the inner and outer retinal layers.[1]

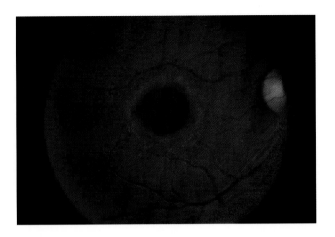

**Figure 5.13** *Traumatic macular hole: note the large diameter (1500 μm) and the surrounding cuff of subretinal fluid.*

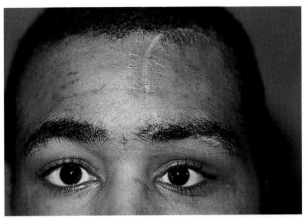

*a*

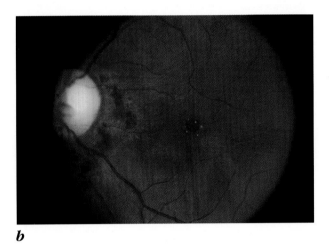

*b*

**Figure 5.14** *Patient with multiple orbital fractures and post-traumatic enophthalmos (A). Fundus examination demonstrates a well demarcated macular hole (B).*

Symptoms include decreased visual acuity and central scotoma. A macular hole typically appears as a round, sharply defined full-thickness defect in the center of the macula with a surrounding cuff of subretinal fluid (Fig. 5.13). Most idiopathic macular holes are 300–500 μm in diameter (one-fifth to one-third disc diameter), but the larger macular holes are often associated with blunt trauma (Fig. 5.14). Fluorescein angiography demonstrates a window defect corresponding to the size of the macular hole which fades in the late frames. Macular holes are stable lesions which rarely are an isolated cause of retinal detachment.[12] Recently, pars plana vitrectomy with fluid gas exchange has been performed for traumatic macular holes, with promising results.[13]

## TRAUMATIC RETINAL DETACHMENT AND ASSOCIATED CONDITIONS

### Retinal detachment

Approximately 10–20% of adult patients with rhegmatogenous retinal detachment report a history of blunt ocular trauma. Traumatic retinal detachment typically occurs in males during the third decade of life. In contrast, nontraumatic retinal detachment characteristically occurs during the sixth decade and has an equal gender distribution.[14] The majority of retinal detachments in children result from ocular trauma.

Trauma includes sudden deformation of the vitreous, and retinal damage may occur in areas of firm vitreoretinal adhesion, such as the fovea, areas of lattice degeneration, chorioretinal scars, and, most significantly, the vitreous base. Retinal damage at the vitreous base may result in vitreous base avulsion, retinal dialysis, peripheral retinal tears, and giant retinal tears. Retinal dialyses account for the majority of traumatic retinal detachments, followed by giant retinal tears, retinal flap tears with adherent vitreous (horseshoe tears), and tears at the edge of lattice degeneration. In contrast, retinal dialyses and giant retinal tears together account for less than 10% of nontraumatic retinal detachment.[14]

Patients with injury to the peripheral retina may be asymptomatic or may note the presence of floaters and/or photopsia. When retinal detachment is present, peripheral visual field loss occurs if the detachment extends posterior to the equator (Fig. 5.15), and visual acuity is reduced with macular involvement.

All patients with a history of ocular trauma should undergo binocular indirect ophthalmoscopy with scleral depression to assess for retinal detachment and associated conditions (after an open globe is ruled out).

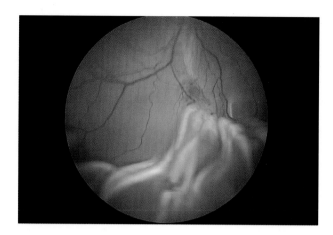

**Figure 5.15** *Symptomatic traumatic retinal detachment.*

## Vitreous base avulsion

Avulsion of the vitreous base from the pars plana and peripheral retina is pathognomonic of blunt ocular trauma. This may occur as an isolated finding or be associated with retinal dialysis or giant retinal tear. Vitreous base avulsion has been reported in up to 26% of patients with traumatic retinal detachment.

Funduscopy reveals an arcuate band elevated over the peripheral retina. When the superior quadrants are involved, the disinserted vitreous base may appear draped over the midperipheral retina (Fig. 5.16). Fragments of pars plana epithelium may occasionally remain adherent to the avulsed vitreous base. Treatment involves cryopexy to the edges to prevent the development of retinal breaks caused by vitreous traction.

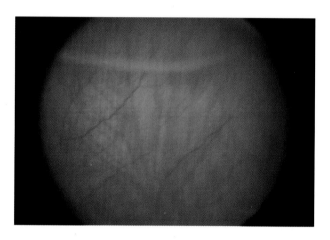

**Figure 5.16** *Avulsed vitreous base appears as a draped, ribbon-like opacity over the superior midperiphery fundus.*

## Retinal dialysis

Retinal dialysis is a separation of the retina from the pars plana epithelium at the ora serrata. This may occur with or without associated retinal detachment. Retinal dialysis appears as a slit at the ora serrata that opens with scleral depression, and serrations within the dialysis are less prominent than normal.[15,16] Retinal detachment, when present, is often localized and minimally elevated, particularly for small or inferior dialyses (Fig. 5.17). Retinal detachments may remain stable or demonstrate slow progression, as formed vitreous often limits the passage of fluid to the subretinal space, and demarcation lines and other signs of chronicity are often present. Retinal dialysis involves the inferotemporal quadrant in 66% of cases. The treatment for retinal dialysis is photocoagulation or cryopexy as prophylaxis for retinal detachment. When retinal detachment is present, scleral buckling surgery is usually indicated.

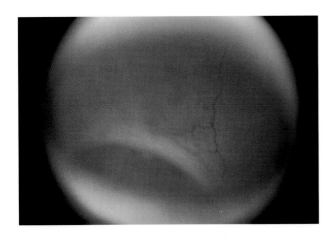

**Figure 5.17** *Retinal dialysis located in the inferotemporal quadrant with an associated localized retinal detachment.*

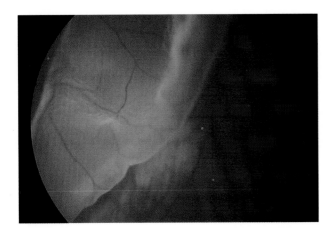

**Figure 5.18** *Giant retinal tear with inverted posterior retinal flap.*

### Retinal tears

Peripheral horseshore-shaped retinal tears and free-floating operculated retinal holes may result from trauma. Trauma induces vitreoretinal traction, and areas of strong vitreoretinal adhesion such as edges of lattice degeneration and chorioretinal scars are especially susceptible. Formed vitreous is attached to the flap of

a horseshoe tear and to the operculum of a free-floating operculated hole, and liquid vitreous may therefore pass through the retinal break to enter the subretinal space. As a result, traumatic retinal tears more often result in retinal detachment compared with retinal dialysis. Occasionally, vitreous hemorrhage is present when a retinal tear involves a torn retinal blood vessel. Treatment for traumatic retinal tears is photocoagulation or cryopexy as prophylaxis for retinal detachment. When retinal detachment is present, scleral buckling procedure is usually performed.

### Giant retinal tears

Giant retinal tears are circumferential peripheral retinal breaks that extend for three or more clock hours. They occur at the posterior edge of the vitreous base and, unlike retinal dialyses, typically result in retinal detachment since liquid vitreous may easily enter the subretinal space. Occasionally, the posterior edge of the tear is folded over the posterior pole (an inverted posterior retinal flap), resulting in poor visualization of the macula (Fig. 5.18). Giant retinal tears are challenging to treat, and management depends on several factors, including the size of the tear, the presence of an inverted posterior retinal flap, and the presence of proliferative vitreoretinopathy. A few giant retinal tears may be treated with scleral buckling surgery. Large tears and tears with an inverted posterior retinal flap are treated with pars plana vitrectomy with fluid gas exchang and placement of a scleral buckle. When proliferative vitreoretinopathy is present, lensectomy may be additionally performed to facilitate removal of anterior vitreous.[16] Perfluorocarbon liquids are often employed intraoperatively to unroll the retina. An extended internal tamponade such as perfluoropropane gas ($C_3F_8$) or silicon oil usually is necessary. The success rate is limited because of recurrent retinal detachment due to the development of proliferative vitreoretinopathy.[17]

### SYSTEMIC TRAUMA WITH POSTERIOR SEGMENT MANIFESTATIONS

A variety of systemic conditions may indirectly affect the eye. Posterior segment manifestations of systemic trauma include Purtscher's retinopathy, Terson's syndrome, Valsalva retinopathy, and shaken baby syndrome.

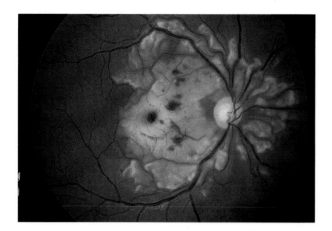

**Figure 5.19** *Purtscher's retinopathy, right eye, showing patches of superficial retinal whitening.*

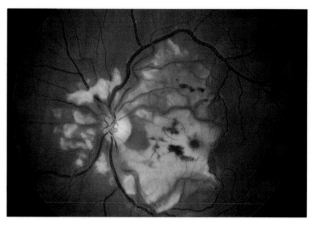

**Figure 5.20** *Purtscher's retinopathy, left eye, same patient as in Fig. 5.19. Note the relatively symmetric involvement.*

## PURTSCHER'S RETINOPATHY

In 1910 Purtscher reported patches of superficial retinal whitening, intraretinal hemorrhages, and papillitis following severe head trauma. The typical setting for Purtscher's retinopathy is severe head trauma in the absence of direct trauma to the globe; however, an indistinguishable fundus appearance may develop in a variety of traumatic injuries and disease (Figs 5.19 and 5.20). These include acute pancreatitis, long bone fracture, compression injuries, air embolization, amniotic fluid embolization, childbirth, hydrostatic pressure syndrome, and connective tissue diseases such as lupus, scleroderma and dermatomyositis.[18]

The condition is typically bilateral, but unilateral cases have been described; in apparent unilateral cases, the fellow eye may demonstrate subtle findings.[19] The fundus findings may be present immediately and may progress for up to 48 hours after the injury. Visual acuity is variable, ranging from 20/20 to count fingers, and an afferent pupillary defect and paracentral scotomas may be present. The course is unpredictable, as some patients experience resolution of visual loss and fundus changes while others develop permanent visual loss associated with macular pigment changes, nerve fiber layer dropout and optic atrophy.[18,19] There is no treatment for Purtscher's retinopathy.

The pathogenesis of fundus findings for all of the aforementioned conditions is uncertain, but multiple emboli may be present in the majority of these conditions. Acute pancreatitis and long bone fracture can lead to arteriolar occlusion from fat embolization, air or amniotic fluid emboli may cause arteriolar occlusion, and complement-induced granulocyte aggregation may result in multiple emboli. Trauma and acute pancreatitis have been shown to activate complement, and complement C5A causes intravascular leukoaggregates. Features of Purtscher's retinopathy that support this concept include sudden onset, multifocal lesions, otherwise healthy retinal vessels, and the characteristic distribution of ischemic patches.[20,21]

## TERSON'S SYNDROME

In 1900 Terson described vitreous hemorrhage in association with intracranial hemorrhage. Subsequently known as Terson's syndrome, intraocular hemorrhage most commonly occurs after subarachnoid hemorrhage, usually resulting from spontaneous rupture of an intracranial aneurysm. Terson's syndrome may also occur after subdural hemorrhage, usually due to trauma.

Fundus findings include vitreous hemorrhage as well as peripapillary preretinal, intraretinal, and/or subretinal hemorrhages (Fig. 5.21). These findings may be unilateral or bilateral. Visual acuity ranges from 20/20 to light perception. Treatment involves observation versus vitrectomy surgery, with ultimate

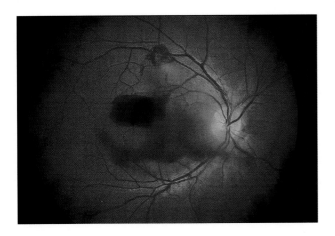

**Figure 5.21** *Terson's syndrome. Preretinal and vitreous hemorrhage.*

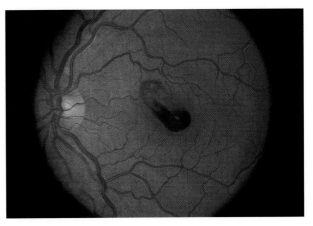

**Figure 5.22** *Valsalva retinopathy. Dumbbell-shaped macular hemorrhage.*

visual outcome 20/50 or better in 83% of eyes. There is usually gradual resolution of the vitreous hemorrhage, but vitrectomy results in more rapid visual recovery. Indications for vitrectomy include young patients in whom early visual rehabilitation may prevent amblyopia, and bilateral Terson's syndrome.[22]

The pathogenesis of Terson's syndrome is controversial. The most accepted mechanism proposes that intracranial hemorrhage produces an acute rise in intracranial pressure that is transmitted within the optic nerve sheath to obstruct the venous drainage from the eye. This acute elevation of venous pressure causes distention and rupture of the fine papillary and retinal capillaries, often resulting in significant hemorrhage. This hemorrhage may spread to the subretinal space, within the retina, the subinternal limiting membrane space, or the vitreous cavity.[23]

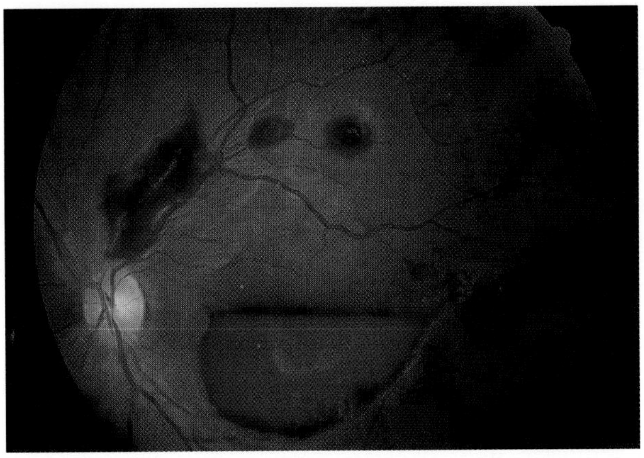

## VALSALVA RETINOPATHY

The Valsalva maneuver is defined as an acute rise of intrathoracic or intra-abdominal pressure against a closed glottis. Incompetent or absent valves in the venous system of the head and neck allow transmission of thoracic or abdominal pressure to result in sudden elevation of ocular venous pressure. In 1972 'Valsalva hemorrhagic retinopathy' was described, resulting from rupture of superficial retinal capillaries. Typical activities producing Valsalva retinopathy include heavy lifting, coughing,

**Figure 5.23** *Valsalva retinopathy. Large preretinal layered macular hemorrhage and peripapillary intraretinal hemorrhages.*

vomiting, sexual activity, and straining during bowel movement. Fundus findings include dumbbell-shaped accumulation of blood in the foveal or parafoveal region and larger round or oval macular hemorrhages (Figs 5.22 and 5.23). The blood is usually located under the internal limiting membrane but it may break through to the subhyaloid space or vitreous cavity. Treatment consists of observation as the hemorrhages eventually resolve and vision returns to normal.[18,24]

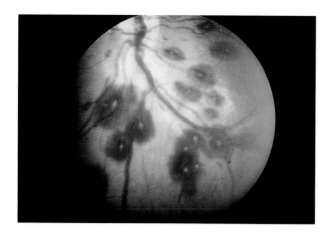

**Figure 5.24** *Presumed shaken baby syndrome. Multiple white-centered intraretinal hemorrhages.*

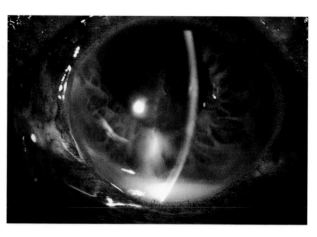

**Fig. 5.25** *Anterior chamber inflammation with hypopyon in a patient with endophthalmitis.*

## SHAKEN BABY SYNDROME

The manual shaking of an infant causes rapid acceleration-deceleration of the head and may result in whiplash-induced ocular manifestations. The typical ophthalmic findings in physically abused children are retinal hemorrhage, cotton-wool spots, and vitreous hemorrhage (Fig. 5.24). In fact, the presence of intraocular hemorrhage should arouse suspicion of possible child abuse in infants with additional injuries. It is important to remember that normal vaginal delivery may result in retinal hemorrhages, although vitreous hemorrhage is extremely uncommon. These retinal hemorrhages may take from weeks to months to resolve. Ocular findings are the presenting signs of child abuse in approximately 5% of cases, and the ophthalmologist may play a critical role in the recognition of this serious condition.[26–28]

## TRAUMATIC ENDOPHTHALMITIS

Endophthalmitis is an uncommon but potentially devastating intraocular infection that often results in severe visual loss. Endophthalmitis is typically classified as either endogenous or exogenous. In endogenous endophthalmitis, the infecting organism spreads to the eye via the bloodstream, whereas in exogenous endophthalmitis, the organism enters the eye from the external environment. Exogenous endoph-

thalmitis is further subdivided into postoperative and post-traumatic endophthalmitis.

Prompt diagnosis of endophthalmitis is essential, since any delay in treatment is detrimental. The most important symptoms are ocular pain and decreased vision, although, in some cases, pain is absent. Signs include purulent discharge, lid edema, conjunctival chemosis and injection, and corneal edema. The most important sign is advanced intraocular inflammation. The anterior chamber reaction is intense and may include circulating cells and flare, fibrinous debris, and/or a hypopyon (Fig. 5.25). In fact, infectious endophthalmitis should be strongly suspected in any patient with a hypopyon. Vitritis is invariably present and may be mild, allowing a view of the retina, or severe, obscuring all retinal details. Additional findings may be present, depending on the clinical situation. (For example, in acute postoperative endophthalmitis following cataract surgery, there may be evidence of wound incompetence or posterior capsular rupture).

Classification of endophthalmitis allows more precise prediction of the infecting organism and may direct treatment. For example, patients who develop endogenous endophthalmitis are typically chronically ill, immunosuppressed, and/or have a known colonized site such as an infected intravenous catheter, endocarditic heart valve, pyelonephritic kidney, or osteomyelitic bone. A wide variety of bacteria and fungi may thus be hematogenously disseminated to the eye from remote sites or from generalized septicemia. Typical gram positive bacteria include Staphylococcus species (cutaneous infec-

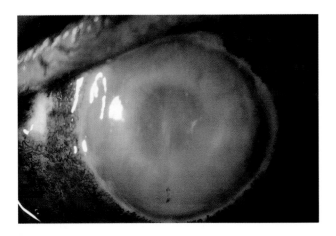

**Fig. 5.26** *Endogenous endophthalmitis. Anterior chamber inflammation with hypopyon in a patient with cutaneous infection from chronis indwelling catheter and Candida endophthalmitis.*

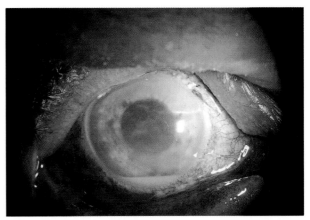

**Fig. 5.27** *Acute postoperative endophthalmitis. Anterior chamber inflammation with hypopyon 2 days following cataract surgery. Cultures grew Staphylococcus epidermidis.*

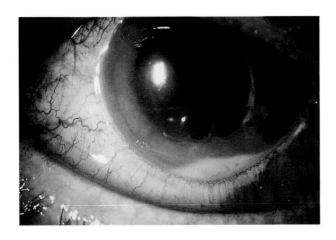

**Fig. 5.28** *Chronic postoperative endophthalmitis. Hypopyon noted 6 months following cataract surgery. Note the absence of severe anterior chamber inflammation. Cultures grew Propionibacterium acnes.*

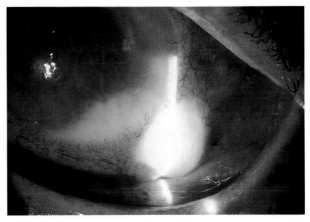

**Fig. 5.29** *Bleb-related endophthalmitis. Streptococcus pneumoniae endophthalmitis 3 years following trabeculectomy surgery for glaucoma. Note the white material filling the entire inferotemporal bleb and the hypopyon.*

tions), Streptococcus species (endocarditis), and Bacillus species (intravenous drug abuse). Gram negative organisms include Neisseria species (meningitis), Hemophilus species, and enterics such as E. coli and Klebsiella. Fungal species include Candida (chronic indwelling catheter often associated with hyperalimentation) (Fig. 5.26) and Aspergillus (intravenous drug abuse).

Similarly, for postoperative endophthalmitis, certain infectious organisms are often associated with certain clinical settings. Postoperative endophthalmitis accounts for approximately 60% of all cases of culture-positive endophthalmitis. Acute postoperative endophthalmitis develops within 1–14 days following intraocular surgery. Mild infections are usually caused by Staphylococcus epidermis (Fig. 5.27) whilse severe inflammation may be caused by Staphylococcus aureus, Streptococcus species, and gram negative organisms such as Pseudomonas and Proteus. Chronic postoperative endophthalmitis

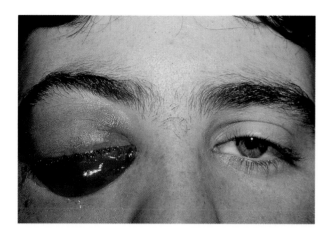

**Fig. 5.30** *Proptosis, periorbital edema, and hemorrhagic chemosis 20 hours following an open globe injury with metallic intraocular foreign body. History revealed hammering metal on metal.*

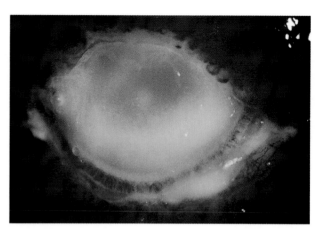

**Fig. 5.31** *Same patient as Fig. 6. Severe intraocular inflammation and corneal ring abscess associated with Bacillus cereus infection.*

occurs two weeks to two years after surgery. Typical organisms include Staphylococcus epidermidis, Propionibacterium acnes (Fig. 5.28), and Candida. One specific type of intraocular surgery deserves special mention: conjunctival filtering blebs for glaucoma. Bacteria, particularly Hemophilus influenzae and Streptococcus pneumoniae (Fig. 5.29), may enter the eye through an intact or leaking conjunctival filtering bleb at any time following this type of glaucoma surgery.

The incidence of traumatic endophthalmitis among all cases of culture-proven endophthalmitis is approximately 25%. Post-traumatic endophthalmitis occurs in 2–8% of eyes following open globe injuries, and it occurs in 7–13% of eyes with a retained intraocular foreign body.[28–30] There are several distinctive features of traumatic endophthalmitis compared with endophthalmitis in other clinical settings: the diagnosis may be more difficult; Bacillus species are likely pathogens; polymicrobial infection is more common; the prognosis is usually very poor.[31]

The diagnosis of traumatic endophthalmitis may be difficult because ocular tissue damage secondary to the trauma may obscure the infectious signs. Media opacities such as corneal edema, intraocular hemorrhage, and/or traumatic cataract may limit the visualization needed to detect signs of endophthalmitis. In addition, trauma has associated sterile inflammation which may be difficult to distinguish from intraocular infection. Since delay in diagnosis may be detrimental, one should suspect endophthalmitis in any open globe injury with unusually severe inflammation, and sterile inflammation should be considered a diagnosis of exclusion. The diagnosis involves the immediate microscopic examination and culture of external discharge, aqueous, and vitreous. The collection technique for these specimens in traumatic endophthalmitis is similar to that for endophthalmitis of any other type. Aqueous fluid is obtained by a needle inserted into the anterior chamber at the limbus. Vitreous fluid is obtained by a needle or vitreous cutter instrument inserted through the pars plana. A vitrectomy may be performed, depending on the severity of the situation. Diagnostic smears should include Gram and Giemsa stains, and additional stains are employed depending on the suspected organism. Typical culture media include blood agar, chocolate agar, liquid thioglycolate media, and Sabouraud's agar.

The most common causative organisms in traumatic endophthalmitis are Bacillus species and Staphylococcus epidermidis, each accounting for approximately 25% of cases. Less likely organisms include Streptococcus species, gram negative organisms, Staphylococcus aureus, and fungal species. Approximately 10% of cases are polymicrobial. Traumatic endophthalmitis is unique in having a high incidence of Bacillus cases and polymicrobial infections. Bacillus cereus is a gram-positive, aerobic,

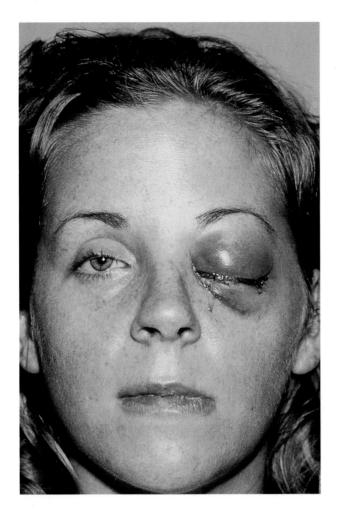

**Fig. 5.32** *Proptosis and periorbital edema associated with Bacillus cereus endophthalmitis.*

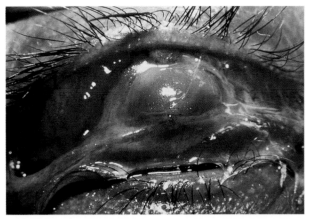

**Fig. 5.33** *Same patient as Fig. 8. Note the marked purulent discharge and severe intraocular inflammation.*

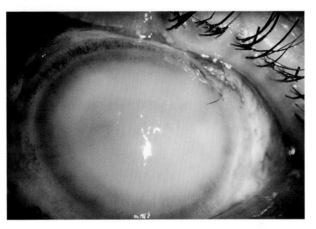

**Fig. 5.34** *Corneal ring abscess and severe intraocular inflammation 30 hours following repair of open globe injury. Cultures grew Bacillus cereus.*

spore forming bacillus that is ubiquitous. It elaborates several enzymes and toxins. The natural habitat of Bacillus cereus is the soil, and farm- and soil-related trauma is particularly associated with Bacillus endophthalmitis.[32,28] Another clinical situation which should alert the clinician to the possibility of Bacillus infection is an open globe injury with a retained intraocular foreign body. Most foreign bodies that enter the eye are potentially contaminated, with either the foreign body itself carrying infectious material, or bringing in material from the eyelid or ocular surface. If the nidus of infectious material is large enough, there is potential for the development of endophthalmitis. Although it is not known how much infectious material is sufficient to cause infec-

tion, the virulence of certain organisms such as Bacillus is high, and traumatic endophthalmitis is most common in injuries with a retained intraocular foreign body[33] (Figs 5.30 and 5.31). The clinical course of Bacillus cereus endophthalmitis is explosive and devastating. Within 24 hours of the injury, patients may develop severe orbital pain, extreme proptosis, periorbital edema, and conjunctival chemosis (Figs 5.32 and 5.33). A distinctive sign of Bacillus infection is a corneal ring abscess associated with peripheral corneal edema[34] (Figs 5.34–5.36). This sign is usually associated with irreversible visual loss. Patients with Bacillus cereus endophthalmitis may also develop constitutional signs such as low-grade fever and a polymorphonuclear leukocytosis.

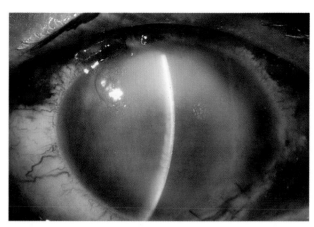

**Fig. 5.36** *Corneal ring abscess and severe intraocular inflammation 48 hours following repair of open globe injury. Cultures grew Bacillus cereus.*

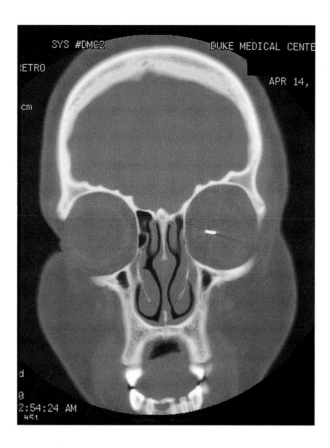

**Fig. 5.35** *Same patient as Fig. 10. CT scan demonstrates retained metallic intraocular foreign body.*

The prognosis of traumatic endophthalmitis is poor, especially when Bacillus cereus is the causative agent. By the time infection is evident clinically, treatment may be insufficient to reverse the infectious process. With severe intraocular inflammation in the presence of a corneal ring abscess, there is almost certain irreversible visual loss. Early recognition and treatment are therefore essential. If signs of endophthalmitis appear in a patient with a recent open globe injury, intravitreal antibiotics should be administered at the time of aqueous and vitreous sampling. The choice of intravitreal antibiotics is controversial, but many practitioners recommend an aminoglycoside such as amikacin with vancomycin and/or clindamycin.[31] These choices continue to be modified by new experimental evidence and clinical experi-

ence. Systemic and topical antibiotics are also recommended. Intravitreal antibiotic therapy is essential because systemic and topical antibiotics may not penetrate the globe in sufficient concentration to eradicate the infection. Since traumatic endophthalmitis is associated with rapid progression and a devastating outcome, some reports advocate the use of prohylactic antibiotics (topical, subconjunctival, intravitreal, and systemic) in the setting of an intraocular foreign body or in an injury associated with dirt or vegetable matter.[31] Most clinicians agree that vitrectomy surgery (with intravitreal antibiotic and, in some cases, intravitreal steroid injection) is indicated for the more severe cases of traumatic endophthalmitis. For injuries associated with intraocular foreign bodies, immediate vitrectomy with foreign body removal is essential. Despite aggressive treatment, the outcome is often poor; final visual acuity was 20/400 or better in only 1 of 17 patients with Bacillus species infection and in 13 of 24 patients with Staphylococcus epidermidis infection, and polymicrobial infections were associated with an even greater degree of visual loss.[31] Consequently, one must always maintain a high index of suspicion for possible endophthalmitis in the setting of ocular trauma, and prophylaxis as well as aggressive treatment of suspected cases are critical.

# REFERENCES

1  Bressler SB, Bressler NM. Traumatic maculopathies. In: Shingleton BJ, Hersh PS, Kenyon KR, eds. *Eye Trauma* (St Louis, MI: Mosby-Year Book, 1991): 187–94.

2  Kelley JS, Dhaliwal RS. Traumatic chorioretinopathies. In: Ryan SJ, ed. *Retina* 2nd edn. (St Louis, MI: Mosby-Year Book, 1994): 1783–96.

3  Hart JCD, Frank HJ. Retinal opacification after blunt nonperforating concussional injuries to the globe; a clinical and retinal fluorescein angiographic study. *Trans Ophthalmol Soc UK* 1975; **95**: 94.

4  Gregor Z, Ryan SJ. Blood–retinal barrier after blunt trauma to the eye. *Graefes Arch Clin Exp Ophthalmol* 1982; **219**: 205–8.

5  Kohno T, Ishibashi T, Inomata H et al. Experimental macular edema of commotio retinae; preliminary report. *Jpn J Ophthalmol* 1983; **27**: 149–56.

6  Pulido JSW, Blair NP. The blood–retinal barrier in Berlin's edema. *Retina* 1987; **7**: 233–6.

7  Mansour AM, Green WR, Hogge C et al. Histopathology of commotio retinae. *Retina* 1992; **12**: 24–8.

8  Aguilar JP, Green WR. Choroidal rupture. A histopathologic study of 47 cases. *Retina* 1984; **4**: 269–75.

9  Martin DF, Ash CC, McCuen BW II et al. Treatment and pathogenesis of traumatic chorioretinal rupture (sclopetaria). *Am J Ophthalmol* 1994; **117**: 190–200.

10  Cox MS, Schepens CL, Freeman HM. Retinal detachment due to ocular contusion. *Arch Ophthalmol* 1966; **76**: 678–85.

11  Gass JDM. Idiopathic senile macular hole. Its early stages and pathogenesis. *Arch Ophthalmol* 1988; **106**: 629–39.

12  Aaberg TM, Blair CJ, Gass JDM. Macular holes. *Am J Ophthalmol* 1970; **69**: 555–62.

13  Glaser BM. Treatment of giant retinal tears combined with proliferative vitreoretinopathy. *Ophthalmology* 1986; **93**: 1193–7.

14  Goffstein R, Burton TC. Differentiating traumatic from non-traumatic retinal detachment. *Ophthalmology* 1982; **89**:361–8.

15  Cox MS, Schepens CL, Freeman HM. Retinal detachment due to ocular contusion. *Arch Ophthalmol* 1966; **76**::678–85.

16  Thompson JT. Traumatic retinal tears and detachments. In: Shingleton BJ, Hersh PS, Kenyon KR, eds. *Eye Trauma* (St Louis, MI: Mosby-Year Book, 1991): 195–203.

17  Billington BM, Leaver PK. Vitrectomy and fluid-silicon oil exchange for giant retinal tears: results at 18 months. *Graefes Arch Clin Exp Ophthalmol* 1986; **224**: 7–10.

18  Gass JDM. *Stereoscopic Atlas of Macular Diseases: Diagnosis and Treatment*, 2nd edn. (St Louis, MI: CV Mosby, 1987).

19  Burton TC. Unilateral Purtscher's retinopathy. *Ophthalmology* 1980; **87**: 1096–105.

20  Blodi BA, Johnson MW, Gass JDM et al. Purtscher's-like retinopathy after childbirth. *Ophthalmology* 1990; **97**: 1654–9.

21  Jacob HS, Goldstein IM, Shapiro I et al. Sudden blindness in acute pancreatitis: possible role of complement-induced retinal leukoembolization. *Arch Intern Med* 1981; **141**: 134.

22  Shultz PN, Sobol WM, Weingeist TA. Long-term visual outcome in Terson's syndrome. *Ophthalmology* 1991; **98**: 1814–9.

23  Weingeist TA, Goldman EJ, Folk JC et al. Terson's syndrome. Clinicopathologic correlations. *Ophthalmology* 1986; **93**: 1435–42.

24  Duane TD. Valsalva hemorrhagic retinopathy. *Trans Am Ophth Soc* 1972; **70**: 298–313.

25  Caffey J. The whiplash shaken infant syndrome: manual shaking by the extremities with whiplash-induced intracranial and intraocular bleedings, linked with residual permanent brain damage and mental retardation. *Pediatrics* 1974; **54**: 396–403.

26  Friendly DS. Ocular manifestations of the physical child abuse. *Trans Am Acad Ophthalmol Otolaryngol* 1971; **75**: 331–2.

27  Harley RD. Ocular manifestations of child abuse. *J Pediatr Ophthalmol Strabismus* 1980; **17**: 5013.28    Affeldt JC, Flynn HW, Forster RK et al. Microbial endophthalmitis resulting from ocular trauma. *Ophthalmology* 1987; **94**:407–13.

29  Brinton GS, Topping TM, Hyndiuk RA et al. Post-traumatic endophthalmitis. *Arch Ophthalmol* 1984; **102**:547–50.

30  Williams DF, Mieler WF, Abrams GW et al. Results and prognostic factors in penetrating ocular injuries with retained intraocular foreign bodies. *Ophthalmology* 1988; **95**:911–16.

31  O'Brien TP, Choi S. Trauma related ocular infections *Ophthalmol Clin North Am* 1995; **8/4**:667–79.

32  Boldt HC, Pulido JS, Blodi CF ewt al. Rural endophthalmitis. *Ophthalmology* 1989; **96**:1722–26.

33  Mieler WF, Ellis MK, Williams DF, Han DP. Retained intraocular foreign bodies and endophthalmitis. *Ophthalmology* 1990; **97**:1532–38.

34  O'Day DM et al. The problem of Bacillus species infection with special emphasis on the virulence of Bacillus cereus. *Ophthalmology* 1981; **88**:833–38.

# *Chapter 6* **Eyelid and lacrimal trauma**

Injury to the eye itself may accompany any injury to the eyelids. Penetrating injuries are more likely to injure the underlying globe (Fig. 6.1); but thermal injuries may involve the globe as well as the eyelids (Fig. 6.2) either by direct damage or by altering the protective barrier with resultant secondary damage to the eye, for example, corneal erosions secondary to incomplete closure. In order to function properly, the eyelids must close completely and a smooth surface (mucous membrane) must lie against the globe. Injury to the eyelids may disturb their function by loss of tissue, displacement secondary to scarring, and contracture leading to incomplete closure and resultant corneal damage (Fig. 6.3). Although much can be accomplished with secondary eyelid repair, the best results are obtained when the eyelids are repaired properly immediately after injury. This region is so vascular that reimplantation of avulsed tissue is quite

feasible and often successful. Composite grafts and free grafts are also practical methods to repair the eyelids. Still the best method of eyelid repair is primary repair, utilizing the tissue available. Repairing a severely injured eyelid may be analogous to solving a complicated jigsaw puzzle (Fig. 6.4). The periocular region may be divided into five separate areas, each with its own distinguishing characteristics and structures (Fig. 6.5). Injuries to the upper eyelid may involve the levator aponeurosis, the lacrimal gland, and the upper canaliculus. Lower eyelid injuries may involve the inferior canaliculus. Medial canthal injuries may involve both canaliculi, the lacrimal sac and the medial canthal tendon. Inadequate repair may result in epiphora and disfigurement. Improperly repaired lateral canthal injuries may result in unsightly and poorly functioning dystopia of the lateral lower lid and canthus (Fig. 6.6).

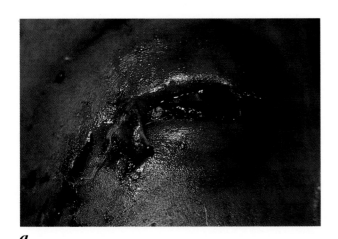

*a*

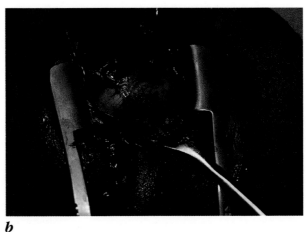

*b*

**Figure 6.1** *Apparent injury to the lower lid and lateral canthus (a). Exploration demonstrates laceration of the globe near the insertion of the lateral rectus (b).*

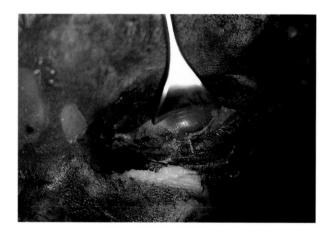

**Figure 6.2** *Severe thermal injury causing full-thickness burns of the eyelids and underlying globe.*

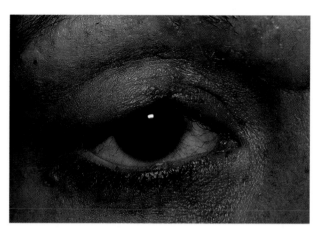

**Figure 6.3** *Eyelid notching caused by inadequate repair and resultant corneal erosion.*

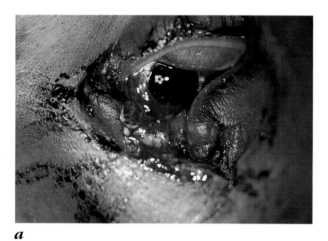

*a*

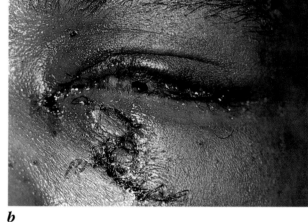

*b*

**Figure 6.4** *Complicated horizontal and vertical lower eyelid laceration (a); appearance after primary repair (b).*

When evaluating periocular injuries, one should think in terms of the structures present in each of these five regions and repair those that are damaged. The most common error in evaluating and treating periorbital injuries is failure to detect and repair injuries to these underlying structures. Another common error is improper repair of the eyelid margin and vertical eyelid laceration, allowing notching and contracture (Fig. 6.3). Even a properly repaired eyelid margin may notch if contracting forces are not neutralized in the postoperative period (Fig. 6.7). These forces may be neutralized by traction sutures, tarsorrhaphy or Oculinum (Botox-Allergan) injections.

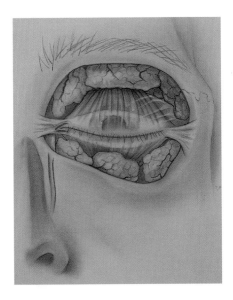

**Figure 6.5** *Periocular region may be divided into five distinct regions: upper eyelid, lower eyelid, medial canthus, lateral canthus, and eyebrow.*

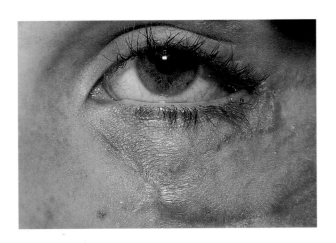

**Figure 6.6** *Inadequate repair of the lateral canthal region resulting in dystopia of the canthus, exacerbated by contraction of a skin graft.*

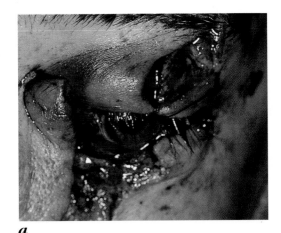

*a*

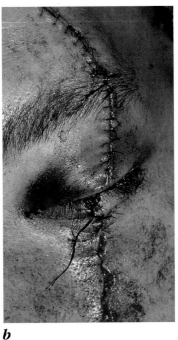

*b*

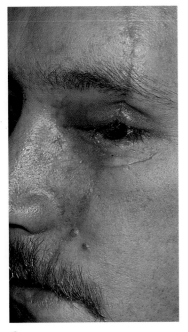

*c*

**Figure 6.7** *Severe vertical lacerations of the upper and lower eyelids (a). Appearance of eyelids with well opposed margins after primary repair (b). Subsequent notching of the upper eyelid due to contraction of scar (c).*

## PRIMARY REPAIR OF THE LOWER EYELID

A simple vertical laceration of the lower eyelid may be repaired in the following manner. If the edges are smooth and well demarcated they can be approximated without removal of tissue. A ragged laceration may be freshened by excising the ragged edges in a pentagonal fashion as one would when excising a full-thinkness eyelid lesion (Fig. 6.8). A 6-0 double-armed silk suture is passed from the severed margin through adjacent Meibomian glands on each side of the laceration. Proper placement of this suture approximates the eyelid margin and is essential for proper alignment. This suture is then placed on upward stretch, exposing the lacerated tarsus. A 6-0 Vicryl suture (Ethicon, Sommerville, NJ) is passed through each side of the tarsus and tied. This approximates the tarsus. Since this represents the strength of the closure, two sutures are usually used. Two additional silk sutures are placed anterior and posterior to the initial marginal suture. These extra sutures help to obviate lid notching and insure proper alignment of the eyelid margin. The vertical closure of the posterior lamella of the eyelid gives it structural integrity. Care should be taken so that the suture or its knots do not rub on the cornea, causing a painful erosion. Closure of the skin–orbicularis layer adds to cosmesis. The author accomplished this with 6-0 mild chromic sutures; however, 6 or 7-0 silk sutures are certainly acceptable. The problem with silk sutures is that they have to be removed postoperatively and if not removed in a timely fashion (5–6 days) unsightly suture tracts may develop. A small skin hook is placed into the wound and tension applied inferiorly. The skin sutures are then placed. Excessive skin is excised in a small triangle as the closure is completed. If there is an accompanying defect in the skin-muscle lamella, this is pieced together like a jigsaw puzzle after the vertical defect has been closed (Fig. 6.9). Anterior lamella defects should not be closed with excessive vertical tension (Fig. 6.10 (a) and (b)) for postoperative ectropion may develop (Fig. 6.10 (c)). If there is too little skin to close the defect without undue tension, a free skin graft may be taken from the retroauricular region. The eyelids are a very vascular region and very accommodating to skin grafting.

What if the defect is too great to close primarily? The next step is to perform a canthotomy/cantholysis to mobilize the lower lid and lateral canthus. This allows closure of a defect involving approximately

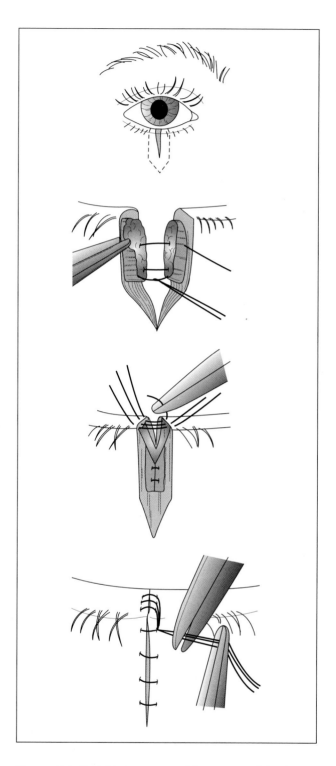

**Figure 6.8** *Full-thickness vertical laceration of the lower eyelid. Placement of a double-armed 6-0 silk suture through Meibomian gland orifices on each side of the laceration. Upward traction is placed on the lid margin while the tarsus is closed with absorbable suture. Final closure of the eyelid margin with 6-0 silk sutures. Care is taken to avoid suture rubbing on the cornea.*

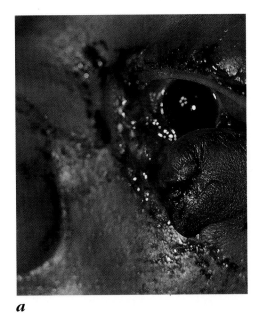

*a*

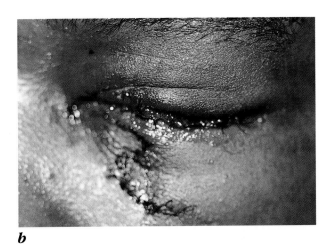

*b*

**Figure 6.9** *Extensive disruption of the anterior lamella (a) may be sutured after the posterior lamella has been repaired.*

**Figure 6.10** *Excessive vertical tension on anterior lamella causing ectropion immediately after repair (a). Lysis of suture obviates the ectropion (b). Tension-free closure of the anterior lamella may necessitate a skin graft (c).*

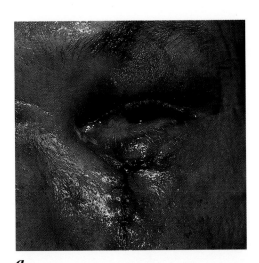

*a*

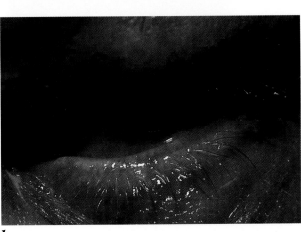

*b*

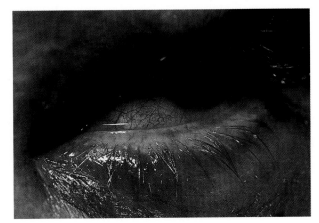

*c*

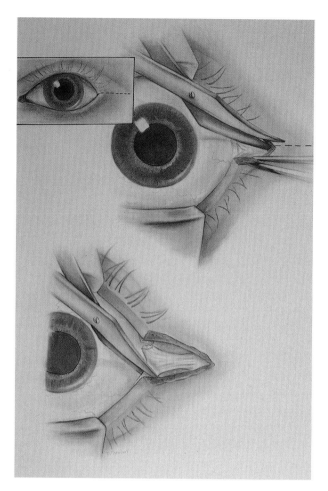

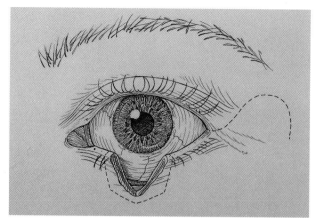

*a*

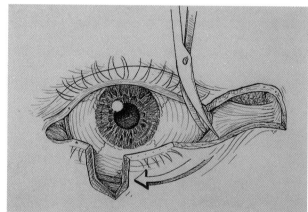

*b*

**Figure 6.11** *Mobilization of the upper or lower eyelid by performing a canthotomy/cantholysis.*

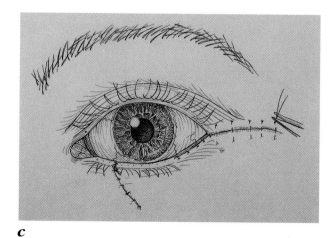

*c*

**Figure 6.12** *Mobilization of the lower eyelid with a sliding Tenzel flap.*

50% of the eyelid in older individuals (Fig. 6.11). If primary closure is still not possible, the lateral canthal region can be mobilized with a sliding skin-muscle flap as described by Tenzel (Fig. 6.12).[1] These procedures may be combined with composite grafts from the uninjured eyelid. As the diagrams indicate, these procedures require an intact lateral eyelid and lateral canthus to mobilize and anastomose with the residual medial eyelid.

The Tenzel flap involves extending the lateral canthotomy incision in a semicircular fashion (Fig. 6.12 (a) and (b)) over the lateral orbital wall and mobilizing a large skin-muscle flap. This allows advancement of the intact lateral lower eyelid and closure of larger defects than may be closed with

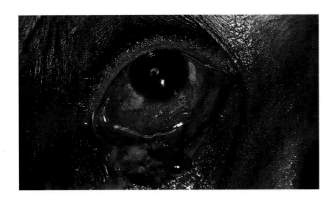

**Figure 6.13** *Large lower eyelid defect requiring a sliding tarsoconjunctival flap for reconstruction.*

canthotomy/cantholysis alone. Conjunctiva from the lateral lower fornix may be mobilized to line the inside of the advancement flap in order to avoid symblepharon formation.

Larger defects involving more than 60% of the eyelid or those involving the lateral eyelid (Fig. 6.13) may be closed with a sliding tarsoconjunctival graft from the upper eyelid. First described by Hughes,[2] and subsequently modified by others, this is a useful procedure for complete reconstruction of the lower eyelid. The posterior lamella (conjunctiva and tarsus) is borrowed from the upper eyelid with its blood supply intact (Fig. 6.14 (b)). A sliding skin muscle advancement flap or a free skin graft provides the anterior lamella (Fig. 14 (c)). Although surrounded by the mystique of oculo-

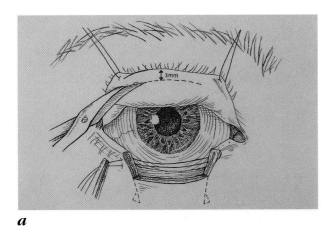

*a*

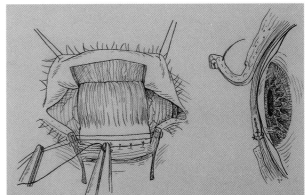

*b*

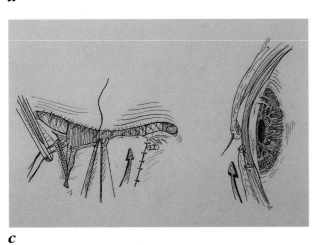

*c*

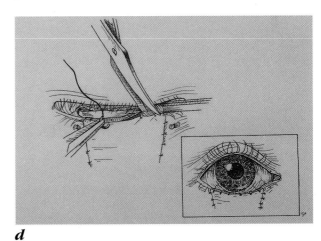

*d*

**Figure 6.14** *Technique for reconstructing lower eyelid with a sliding tarsoconjunctival flap from the upper eyelid (Hughes procedure). Lower eyelid defect is approximated with 4-0 silk sutures (a). Upper eyelid is everted and incised 3-4 mm from the eyelid margin (a). A tarsoconjunctival flap is advanced and sutured into the lower eyelid defect (b). A skin-muscle flap is advanced from beneath the lower eyelid to cover the tarsoconjunctival flap. A free skin graft may be substituted if adequate skin is not available (c). Four to six weeks later the tarsoconjunctival flap may be lysed and the reconstructed eyelid opened (d).*

plastic surgery, this is not a difficult procedure to perform, with good cosmetic and functional results obtainable if a few rules are followed.

## TECHNIQUE

The upper eyelid and remnant of the lower eyelid is copiously infiltrated with an anesthetic solution containing an equal combination of lidocaine with epinephrine and bupivacaine with epinephrine. An ampule of hyaluronidase is added to the solution. A 4-0 silk suture is placed through the margin of the upper eyelid and it is inverted. The initial incision through the conjunctiva and tarsus must be made 3–4 mm from the eyelid margin to avoid notching of the eyelid (Fig. 6.14 (a)). The incision extends through the tarsus. The horizontal length of the incision is determined by measuring the horizontal defect in the lower eyelid that needs to be filled. This is done by placing a 4-0 silk suture through both ends of the defect, tightening it to place the severed ends on mild tension and then measuring, with a caliper, the space needing to be filled (Fig. 6.14(a)). This is the other key maneuver. If tension is not placed upon the defect, the tarsoconjunctival graft will be too large and an ectropion will result postoperatively.

After horizontally incising the tarsoconjunctival graft to fit the defect, the vertical edges of the graft are incised and extended the vertical width of the tarsus. Dissection is accomplished with sharp Wescott scissors (Stortz, St Louis, MO) and the tarsus is easily dissected from the overlying pretarsal orbicularis and levator aponeurosis (Fig. 6.14 (b)). At the superior boundary of the tarsus, dissection is continued in the place between Muller's muscle and the levator aponeurosis. This gives the tarsoconjunctival graft a vascular pedicle consisting of conjunctiva and Muller's muscle. This flap is advanced into the lower lid defect and secured with 5 or 6-0 Vicryl sutures (Fig. 6.14 (b)). The tarsoconjunctival graft from the upper eyelid becomes the posterior lamella (tarsus and conjunctiva) of the reconstructed lower eyelid. If the entire lateral lower lid has been lost, the lateral portion of the tarsoconjunctival flap may be secured to the periorbital of the lateral orbital rim with nonabsorbable sutures (Prolene). This reconstructs the lateral canthus and the lateral canthal angle.

After the tarsoconjunctival advancement flap is sutured into position with multiple interrupted sutures, the anterior lamella is reconstructed. Since the tarso-

conjunctival flap has a blood supply, a free retroauricular skin graft may be used; but it is usually more expedient to advance a skin-muscle flap from below the defect (Fig. 6.14 (c)). The advancement flap is sutured to the adjacent lower lid with 6-0 silk sutures, and to the tarsoconjunctival flap with 6-0 Vicryl sutures at what will be the superior edge of the lower lid.

The modified Hughes procedure for total reconstruction of the lower eyelid is very effective for defects with a vertical length of less than one centimeter. It does require occlusion of the involved eye for up to 6 weeks but, in reality, the flap may be severed in 3–4 weeks (Fig. 6.14 (d)). Techniques have also been described for fenestrating the advancement flap to allow the patient to see and the doctor to examine the eye.

## COMPLICATIONS OF LOWER EYELID REPAIR

Ectropion caused by contracture of the repaired anterior lamella of the eyelid may be avoided by not placing vertical tension on the wound and advancing tissue in a horizontal plane (Fig. 6.10). A small retroauricular skin graft, placed primarily, may avoid more difficult reconstruction later. Notching and mild ectropion of the lower eyelid may be treated with release of the contacted scar by multiple Z-plasties or full-thickness retroauricular skin grafting after excision of the contracted tissue.

Notching of the repaired eyelid margin may occur from faulty surgical technique: not aligning the edges properly, failure to place adequate sutures through tarsus, or postoperative contraction of the eyelid. Applying upward stretch to the eyelid, using a traction suture straddling the laceration site may be helpful. The author prefers 4-0 silk over a cotton bolster. The eyelid may also be partially immobilized by injecting Oculinum around the repaired region postoperatively.

## LATERAL CANTHUS

Injury to the lateral eyelid may result in unsightly and dysfunctional lateral canthal laxity. This is exacerbated by gravity and the cicatrizing forces of scarring (Fig. 6.6). The lateral canthal tendon when severed needs to be reattached to the periosteum overlying

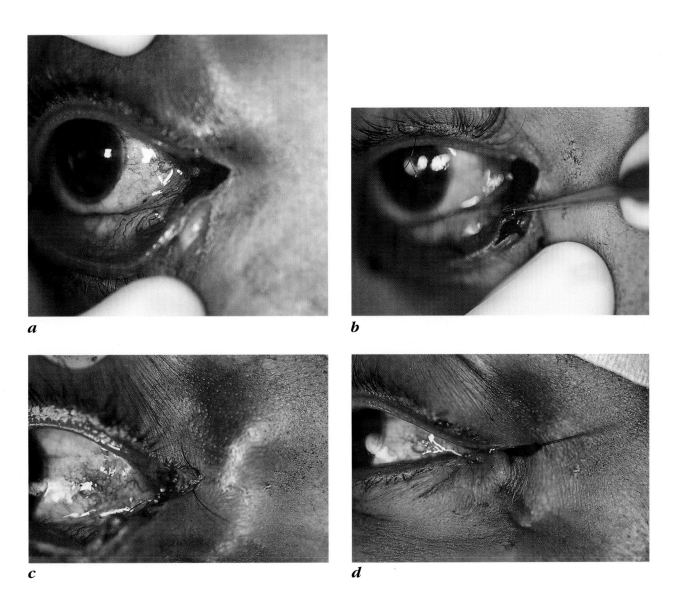

*a*

*b*

*c*

*d*

**Figure 6.15** *Detached lateral canthus repaired by mobilizing a strip of tarsoconjunctiva and reattaching it to the lateral orbital wall with a nonabsorbable suture.*

the lateral orbital tubercle. If this is not done primarily it may be accomplished with a tarsal strip procedure at a later date.[3,4] The lateral canthal angle needs to be overcorrected when tightened to overcome the forces of gravity and cicatrization.

## TARSAL STRIP

If the lateral canthal tendon has been disinserted from the lateral orbital rim, it may be reapproximated by the same technique utilized for tightening the lower eyelid in patients with lower eyelid laxity. A canthotomy and cantholysis is performed as described previously. The severed end of the lower eyelid is split into an anterior lamella containing skin and orbicularis and a posterior lamella of tarsus and conjunctiva (Fig. 6.15 (b)). The conjunctiva is scraped from the posterior lamella with a no. 15 blade. The strip of tarsus is then approximated to the lateral orbital wall at the level of the lateral orbital tubercle. This is accomplished with 5-0 polypropylene suture with an OPS needle (Ethicon,

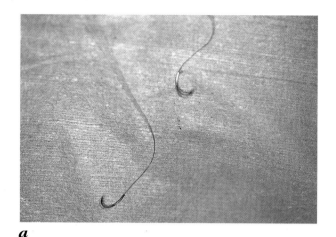

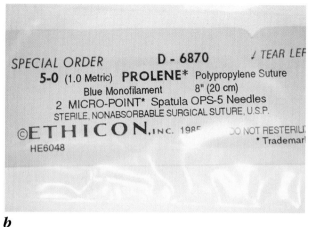

*a*                                    *b*

**Figure 6.16** *A 5-0 polypropylene suture with a sturdy OPS needle (a) available on special order (b).*

Sommerville, NJ) (Fig. 6.16). Both arms of the suture are passed through the tarsal strip from the posterior to the anterior surface (Fig. 6.15 (c)). These are then tied to prevent the suture from 'cheese-wiring' through the tarsus. The tarsal strip is then approximated to the lateral orbital rim. The key maneuver is to pass the needles deep inside the orbital rim to engage the periorbita on the inner surface of the orbital rim. This allows the lid to be firmly approximated to the globe (Fig. 6.15(d)). Once the eyelid is in good apposition to the globe, a second suture is added to reinforce the repair. The skin-muscle flap is then trimmed and the wound closed.

## MEDIAL CANTHUS

Injuries to the medial eyelid and/or the medial canthus may involve the medial canthal tendon, canaliculi, lacrimal sac or nasolacrimal duct (Fig. 6.17).[5] If the medial canthal tendon is severed and not repaired, and unsightly, dysfunctional, traumatic telecanthus results (Fig. 6.18). Medial canthal tendon injury should be suspected in any injury to the medial canthus or mid-face and may be detected by pulling the lower eyelid laterally while palpating the medial canthus. One can feel the tension on an intact medial

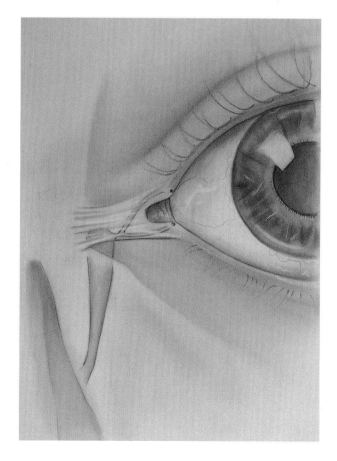

**Figure 6.17** *Medial canthus containing medial canthal tendon, lacrimal sac and canaliculi.*

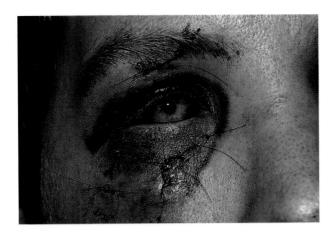

**Figure 6.18** *Traumatic telecanthus resulting from failure to reconstruct the medial canthal tendon at the time of primary repair.*

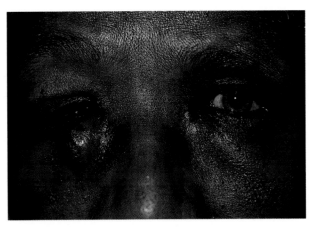

**Figure 6.19** *Bilateral dacryocystitis as a late sequela of a mid-face fracture damaging both nasolacrimal ducts.*

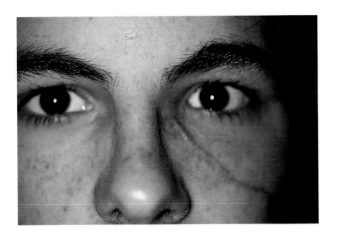

**Figure 6.20** *Facial laceration damaging the lacrimal sac but sparing the canaliculi. Dacryocystorhinostomy resolved the epiphora.*

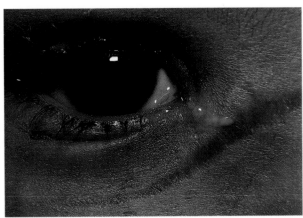

**Figure 6.21** *Neglected facial laceration damaging the lower canaliculus causing intractable epiphora, requiring a conjunctivo dacryocystorhinostomy (cDRC).*

canthal tendon, while, if disinserted, the lower eyelid is easily displaced laterally. A disinserted or severed medial canthal tendon may be primarily repaired or reapproximated to the periosteum with a 5-0 Prolene suture. More extensive disruption, as with mid-face fractures, may require miniplate fixation to the naso-ethmoid complex (see Chapter 10).

Injuries to the lacrimal sac and nasolacrimal duct may result in fistula formation and recurrent dacry-ocystitis (Fig. 6.19 and 6.20). These are easily managed secondarily by performing a dacryocys-torhinostomy (DCR). However, undetected and subsequently unrepaired injuries to the canaliculi may result in intractable epiphora that may be very difficult to manage secondarily with a conjunctival dacryocystorhinostomy (cDCR) (Fig. 6.21). The best treatment for lacerated canaliculi (Figs 6.22 and 6.23) is primary repair with bicanalicular intubation.

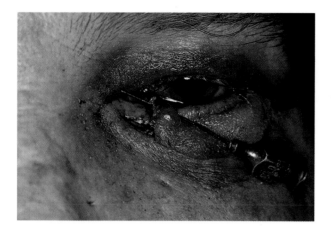

**Figure 6.22** *Simple canalicular laceration of lower eyelid.*

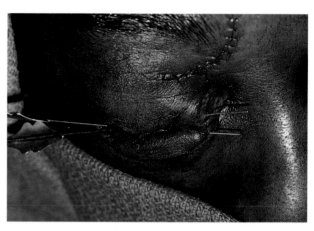

**Figure 6.23** *Bicanalicular laceration.*

## TECHNIQUE OF CANALICULAR REPAIR

The most important issue in evaluating a medial canthal injury is suspecting and detecting injury to the canalicular system.[6] Undetected injury to the lacrimal sac or duct can be effectively managed at a later date by performing a DCR. Late canalicular repair, although described, is usually unsuccessful, and these patients undergo numerous cDCRs with Pyrex tube placement. The tubes extrude recurrently, and the patients are subjected to numerous surgical procedures.

There is no question that there are some canaliculi that cannot be repaired; however, most can be. Prior to repair the severed ends must be found. This can be facilitated with a drop or two of 10% phenylephirine applied to the wound. This constricts the blood vessels, obviates bleeding, and allows better examination of the wound. The illumination and magnification provided by the operating microscope are very helpful in identifying severed ends of canaliculi. A canaliculus lacerated in the eyelid is relatively easy to repair (Fig. 6.24). The proximal and distal ends are identified, and a Crawford probe (Jed-med, St Louis, MO) with sialastic tubing is inserted into the punctal end of the lacerated lid, passed through one end of the lacerated canaliculus, and into the distal canaliculus. The probe is then passed into the lacrimal sac. As bony resistance is encountered, the probe is withdrawn slightly, rotated 90°, and passed down the nasolacrimal duct into the nose. The balled end of the Crawford probe may be hooked with a specially designed hook beneath the inferior turbinate and dragged out of the nares. The other probe is then passed through the uninjured canaliculus, into the lacrimal sac, down the nasolacrimal duct and grasped beneath the inferior turbinate in a similar fashion. Both the injured and the normal canaliculi are now intubated with a loop of sialastic tubing with the free ends exciting the nose. At the conclusion of the procedure the two ends of the sialastic tubing may be tied in a square knot and released into the nose. This allows easy removal at a later date by cutting the closed loop at the medial canthus and extracting the tubing through the punctum.

There are several lacrimal intubation systems commercially available. The Crawford system (Fig. 6.25) is, in the author's experience, the easiest to use, both for the experienced surgeon and the resident-in-training. There are two basic pitfalls encountered with Crawford tube intubation of the lacrimal system. First, not passing the hook along the floor of the nose under the inferior turbinate. It is easy for the occasional nasal surgeon to become disoriented and pass the hook under the middle turbinate or just above the inferior turbinate instead of below it. Subsequent manipulations in this very vascular area result in copious bleeding and obscuration of the surgical field.

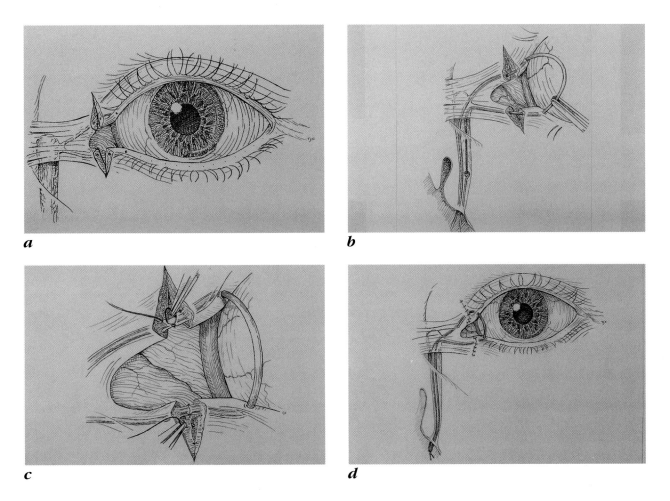

*a*  *b*

*c*  *d*

**Figure 6.24** *Technique for repairing a bicanalicular laceration (a). The lacerated canaliculi are intubated with sialastic tubing and the ends retrieved from the nose with a Crawford hook (b). The lacerated ends are microsurgically anastomosed (c) and the superficial laceration closed.*

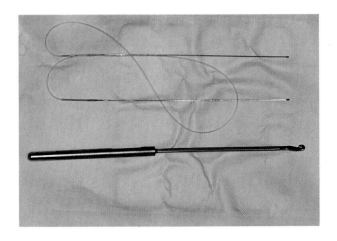

**Figure 6.25** *Crawford canalicular intubation system.*

When this happens (and it will happen) stop manipulation, pack the nose with Afrinized cottonoids and wait 5 minutes. The bleeding will stop. Pass the hook along the floor of the nose, under the inferior turbinate, with the open end of the hook facing superiorly. Beneath the turbinate, rotate the hook 90° medially and slowly extract it from the nose; with the opposite hand, feel for metal-on-metal contact with the probe. When contact is made, withdraw the hook and the probe from the nose. If metal-on-metal contact cannot be felt, a false passage of the probe has been made. Withdraw the probe and reintubate the lacerated canaliculus making certain that the probe is passed down the nasolacrimal duct. Repeat step one above and withdraw the probe and tubing from the nose. The

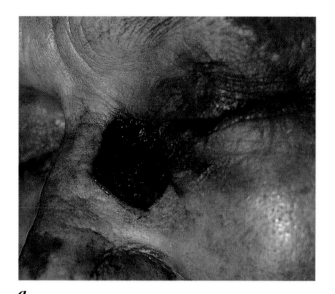

*a*

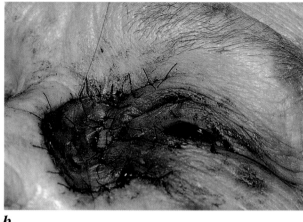

*b*

**Figure 6.26** *Repair of a superficial medial canthal defect with a combination of sliding flaps and a free skin graft.*

lacerated canaliculus may now be microsurgically anastomosed using 8-0 absorbable suture or 10-0 nylon suture. It probably makes no major difference to the final, functional result whether the cut ends of the canaliculus are sutured together or just approximated with the sialastic tubing. The important factor is intubating the canaliculus with the sialastic tubing and allowing it to stent the canaliculus for a least 6–8 weeks. Reapproximation of tarsus to the medial canthal tendon with a 5-0 Vicryl suture lends strength to the closure and supports the canalicular repair.

Arguments have been made against intubating a normal canaliculus and techniques of monocanalicular intubation have been described. In the author's experience monocanalicular intubation does not last long enough to allow appropriate healing of the lacerated canaliculus. These stents may be pulled out or irritate the cornea. It is also very difficult to injure the normal canaliculus by intubating it with a Crawford probe and tubing. The greatest argument against bicanalicular intubation is that the average ophthalmologist is uncomfortable retrieving these probes in the nose and will resort to almost any excuse or rationalization to avoid this discomfort. Retrieving probes from the nose is facilitated by prior cocainization or Afrinization of the nasal mucosa. Constricting the mucosa greatly facilitates work in the nose. To reiterate, pass the Crawford hook flush against the floor of the nose with the open end above. Under the inferior turbinate, rotate the hook

90° medially and slowly withdraw the hook. Contact between hook and probe can be felt and the probe may be gently drawn from the nose. With a little practice this is not a difficult procedure.

Every effort should be made to find and repair the injured canaliculi. Irreparably damaged canalicular systems or neglected injuries will necessitate a cDCR to bypass the injured canalicular system with a Pyrex glass tube. These patients require lifelong follow-up and replacement of their tubes. If at all possible, primary repair, even if delayed 24–48 hours is a much better alternative.

What can be done if the nasal end of the lacerated canaliculus cannot be found? The lacrimal sac may be isolated via a DCR incision, opened and the canaliculi probed from inside the sac outward. The eyelid ends of the canaliculi may be intubated and anastomosed directly to the lacrimal sac. A DCR may then be performed bypassing the nasolacrimal duct and obviating retrieving the probes from the nose.

## MEDIAL CANTHAL INJURIES

If there is no injury to the medial canthal tendon or the nasolacrimal excretory system, medial canthal injuries may be repaired with a combination of sliding skin-muscle flaps from the adjacent upper and

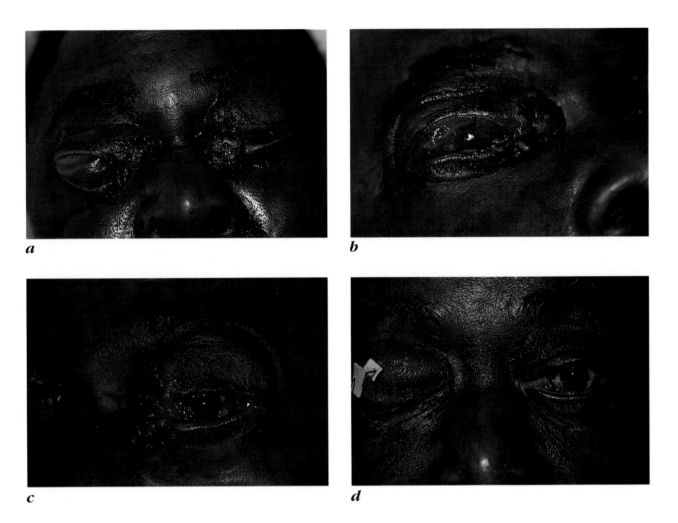

**Figure 6.27** *Pistol-whip injury to face and eyelids with resultant lacerations of both upper eyelids ((a)–(c)). Total ptosis of the right upper eyelid due to irreparably damaged levator muscle (d).*

lower eyelids, with a free skin graft as necessary (Fig. 6.26). These wounds, if untreated, may also heal by granulation—albeit taking much longer—in a cosmetically and functionally acceptable fashion.

## UPPER EYELID

Injuries to the upper eyelid are potentially more complicated than those of the lower eyelid (Fig. 6.27). The inner surface of the upper eyelid constantly rubs against the globe. Any irregularities

secondary to injury or repair, or sutures penetrating the conjunctival surface may cause significant ocular irritation and corneal erosion with the potential for infection. The upper eyelid also contains the levator muscle and its aponeurosis. Undetected trauma to the levator muscle results in an eyelid that is closed or partially closed (Fig 6.27). The lacrimal gland lies in the superior temporal quadrant of the upper eyelid and may be injured concomitantly or during repair of the upper eyelid injury. The upper eyelid is not as forgiving as the lower eyelid. Vertical lacerations of the upper eyelid (Fig. 6.28) may be closed primarily as described for lower eyelid lacerations. Full-thickness sutures through tarsus must not penetrate the

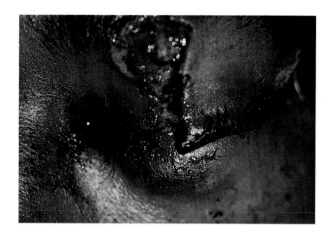

**Figure 6.28** *Full-thickness vertical laceration of the upper eyelid.*

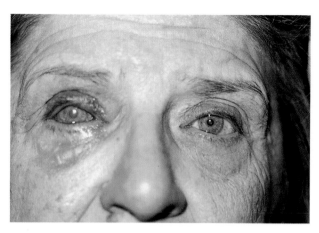

**Figure 6.29** *Suture keratopathy secondary to full-thickness suture through the conjunctiva of the upper eyelid.*

conjunctiva or a suture keratopathy will develop (Fig. 6.29). The lid should be everted after the repair to ensure that the tarsal sutures were not placed through the full thickness of the eyelid. The marginal sutures should be left long and tied over the skin surface of the eyelid to ensure that the knots will not erode the cornea.

If it is necessary to excise a pentagon of upper eyelid to freshen a defect, the parallel sides of the pentagon should be extended the entire vertical width of the tarsus. The apex of the pentagon contains full-thickness supratarsal structures (Fig. 6.30). Attempting to confine the pentagonal excision to the tarsus will result in a cosmetically and functionally unacceptable lid notch. Lid notching may result from faulty marginal eyelid closure, with or without scar contraction. An upper lid notch (Fig. 6.31 (b)) results in incomplete closure of the eyelid and resultant corneal exposure and irritation (Fig. 6.32 (a)). Lid notching may be avoided by careful repair of vertical lacerations and utilizing traction sutures as necessary.

Horizontal lacerations of the upper eyelid may partially or totally transect the levator muscle or aponeurosis causing or partial ptosis (Fig. 6.32 (a)). Lacerations need to be meticulously inspected to detect injury to the levator (Fig. 6.32 (b)). Even in a terribly injured upper eyelid, the levator aponeurosis lies deep to the preaponeurotic fat and often maintains its glistening appearance. The lacerated

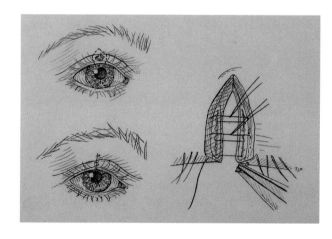

**Figure 6.30** *Proper technique for closure of a vertical upper eyelid laceration: extends the laceration along the entire vertical length of the tarsus and excises supratarsal structures at the apex of the pentagon.*

ends of the levator may be identified and repaired with a nonabsorbable suture (Fig 6.32 (c)). Use of a polypropylene suture facilitates identification of the levator aponeurosis if a subsequent operation is necessary to repair a post-traumatic ptosis.

The lacrimal gland and its ductules may be injured along with the lateral upper eyelid and levator

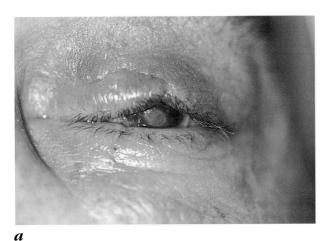
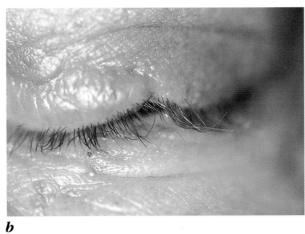

*a*                                          *b*

**Figure 6.31** *Chronically irritated cornea secondary to a notched upper eyelid (b) after faulty repair. Treatment consists of full-thickness excision of the notched eyelid followed by proper repair.*

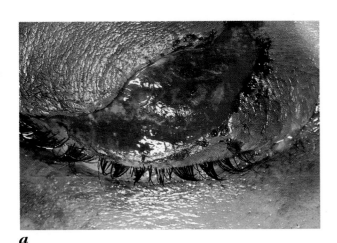
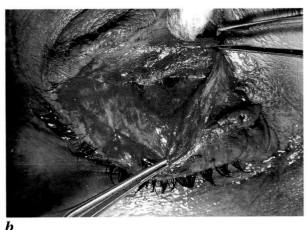

*a*                                          *b*

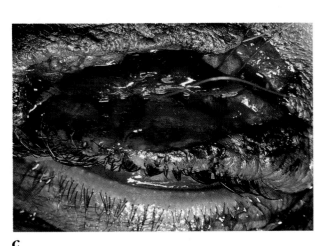

**Figure 6.32** *Horizontal laceration of the upper eyelid (a). Exploration reveals disinsertion of the levator aponeurosis (b), upper forceps from tarsus (lower forceps). Reapproximation of levator to tarsus with a polypropylene suture (c). Note the preaponeurotic fat lying anterior to the levator aponeurosis.*

*c*

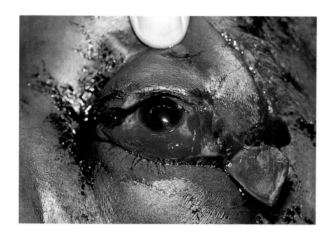

**Figure 6.33** *Knife injury to the lateral upper eyelid and lacrimal gland.*

aponeurosis (Fig. 6.33). The levator aponeurosis divides the lacrimal gland into orbital and palpebral lobes (Fig. 6.5). Injury to the orbital lobe is usually well tolerated and if prolapsed it can be easily repositioned in the lacrimal fossa with a double-armed suture passed through the gland and both arms of the suture passed through the periorbita lining the lacrimal fossa.[7] Denervation of the orbital lobe deprives the palpebral lobe of its parasympathetic innervation with resultant dysfunction. Injury to the palpebral lobe of the lacrimal gland and its ductules may cause or exacerbate a dry eye.

Once the canaliculus, the levator, and the lacrimal gland have been evaluated and attended to, and the vertical laceration repaired, the horizontal component of the laceration may be repaired. This is often similar to putting together a jigsaw puzzle. (Figs 6.34 and

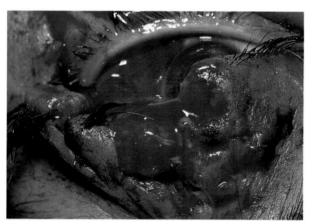

*a*

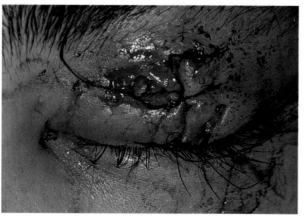

*c*

*b*

**Figure 6.34** *Surgeon's view of a severe horizontal and vertical laceration of the upper eyelid (a). After the vertical component is repaired (b), the horizontal component is pieced together like a jigsaw puzzle (c).*

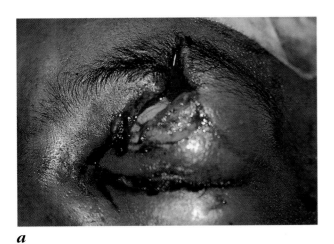
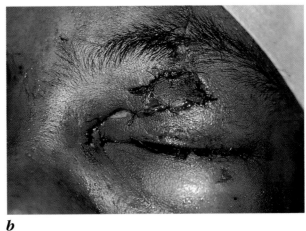

*a*      *b*

**Figure 6.35** *Complex laceration involving the upper eyelid, canaliculus and eyebrow (a). After the canaliculus is repaired and the brow approximated, a skin graft may be utilized to fill the horizontal defect (b).*

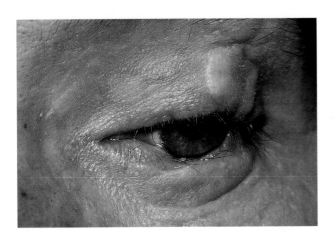

grafts must be meticulously thinned, carefully sutured and splinted with a patch for 5–7 days to obtain the best possible result and avoid unsightly, poorly functioning upper-lid grafts (Fig. 6.36). Some horizontal lacerations with minimal skin loss (Fig. 6.37 (a)) may be left to granulate with a reasonable cosmetic and functional result (Fig. 6.37 (b)–(e)). This may be preferable to skin grafting in some instances.

## LARGE UPPER EYELID LACERATIONS

**Figure 6.36** *Dysfunctional upper eyelid due to a thick and unsightly skin graft.*

6.35). Upper eyelid skin should be conserved whenever possible for the upper eyelid is much less forgiving of skin grafting than the lower eyelid. If skin grafting is absolutely necessary, a graft may be taken from the opposite upper lid. This is the best match; but it must be taken with care so as not to cause retraction and incomplete closure of the normal eyelid. Older patients with redundant lid skin are more suitable than younger patients. These patients may be better grafted with retroauricular skin. These

A large vertical laceration of the upper eyelid may not close primarily. The upper eyelid may be mobilized in a similar fashion to the lower eyelid. First, by performing a canthotomy and cantholysis (Fig. 6.38). If this does not result in sufficient laxity to anastomose the lacerated ends, further mobilization may be attained by advancing a musculocutaneous flap from the lateral orbital region (Fig. 6.39) in a similar fashion to that described for lower eyelid repair. Total loss of the upper eyelid (Fig. 6.40) may tax the ingenuity of an experienced oculoplastic surgeon. Mobilization of a bridge flap, using a portion of the lower eyelid to reconstruct the upper eyelid, is suggested. These results are rarely as satisfying as those obtained in lower eyelid reconstruction (Fig. 6.41).[8]

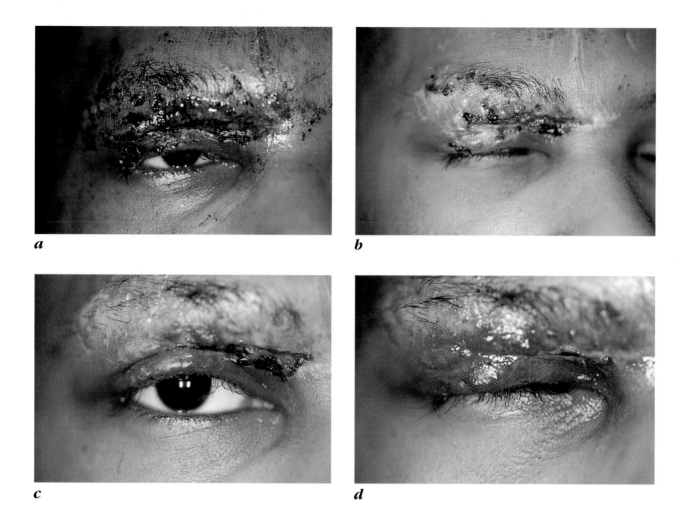

*a*

*b*

*c*

*d*

**Figure 6.37** *A horizontal upper eyelid laceration with avulsion of eyelid skin (a). Sequence of monthly photos ((b), (c)) demonstrating slow healing by secondary intention with an acceptable cosmetic and functional result ((d), (e)).*

*e*

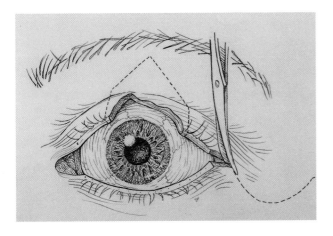

**Figure 6.38** *Mobilization of the upper eyelid by performing a canthotomy and cantholysis.*

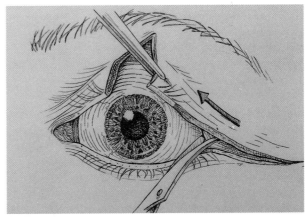

**Figure 6.39** *Further mobilization may be obtained by undermining adjacent tissue and advancing a myocutaneous flap.*

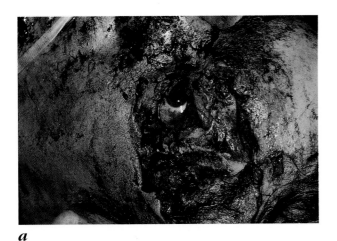

*a*

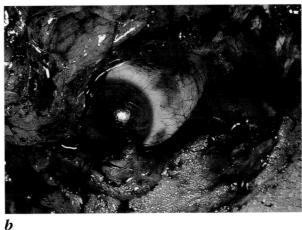

*b*

**Figure 6.40** *Total avulsion and loss of the upper eyelid and partial loss of the lower eyelid due to an automobile accident. Visual acuity was 20/20 and the eye was undamaged.*

## MISCELLANEOUS EYELID INJURIES

### HUMAN BITES

The human bite is still one of the most contaminated wounds that we are called upon to treat. These wounds are often inflicted to the upper eyelid during fights or in a fit of passion (Fig. 6.42). These eyelids are not closed primarily unless they are totally severed or disrupted. They are loosely approximated and treated with a course of intravenous antibiotics. Injuries as shown in Fig. 6.42 are copiously irrigated with saline and Betadine solution and treated with intravenous antibiotics, specifically intravenous cefoxitin 1 g every 8 hours or Augmentin (co-amoxiclav) 500 mg every 8 hours. Even the excellent vascular supply to the eyelids does not make them immune to infection from these very contaminated injuries.[9]

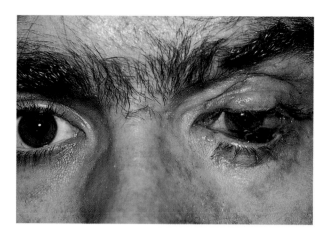

**Figure 6.41** *Patient in Fig. 40 after multiple reconstructive procedures.*

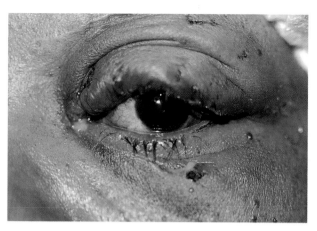

**Figure 6.42** *Human bite to the upper eyelid with minimal disruption of tissue.*

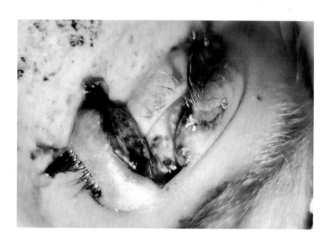

**Figure 6.43** *Partial avulsion of the upper eyelid due to a dog bite. These lids may be primarily repaired after copious irrigation and cleansing.*

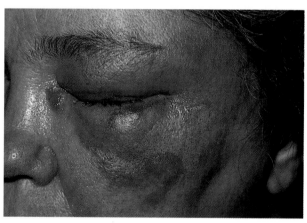

**Figure 6.44** *Scald burn to the eyelids. These partial-thickness burns spare the underlying eye.*

## ANIMAL BITES

Dog bites to the face often occur when a child is playing with a somewhat familiar dog. The distinctive appearance is one bite in the medial canthal region (lower jaw) and another bite in the brow or forehead (upper jaw).[10,11] The lids may be avulsed from the canthus, the trochlea, or medial canthal tendon and the canalicular system may be involved or spared (Fig. 6.43). The surgeon needs to identify the involved structures, repairing them as described previously. Effort should be made to find avulsed eyelid tissue. Totally avulsed eyelids can be re-attached with excellent success.[11] The author treats

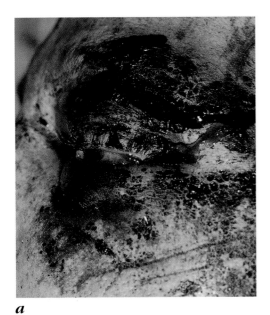

*a*

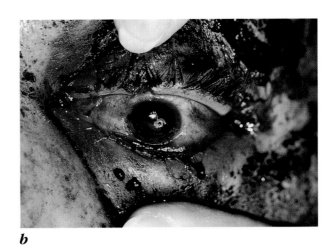

*b*

**Figure 6.45** *Scalding water burn to the face and eyelids (a). The only ocular involvement is a superficial burn to the corneal epithelium (b).*

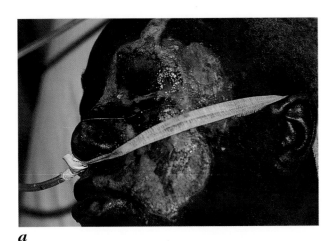

*a*

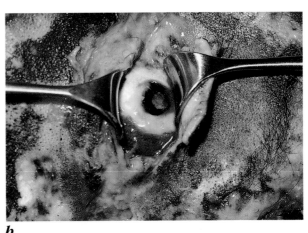

*b*

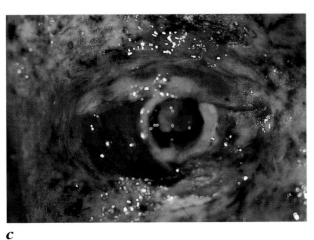

*c*

**Figure 6.46** *Severe contact burn to the face and eyelids ((a), (b)) destroying the patient's only sighted eye (c). Inebriated patient fell asleep on a radiator.*

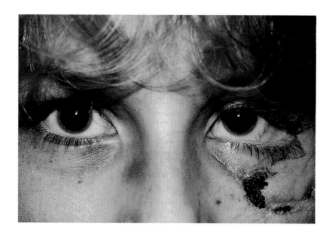

**Figure 6.47** *Extrinsic ectropion caused by scarring and contraction of the tissue adjacent to the eyelid.*

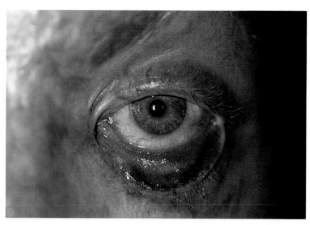

**Figure 6.48** *Intrinsic ectropion caused by injury and contracture of the thin eyelid skin.*

these children with prophylactic antibiotics, specifically penicillin or ampicillin 250–500 mg every 6 hours. Augmentin (co-amoxiclav) 250–500 mg every 8 hours is also appropriate.

## BURNS

The majority of eyelid burns are superficial, partial thickness injuries, sparing the underlying eye and healing within one week (Fig. 6.44).[12,13] There is no good treatment for full-thickness eyelid burns. Usually the underlying eye is spared (Fig. 6.45), but in exceptional cases, usually contact burns, it may also be destroyed (Fig. 6.46). Treatment should entail attempts to protect and save the eye.

Initially after injury the eyelids are swollen and the globe protected by the swollen lids (Fig. 6.44 and 6.45). The eye should be carefully examined as soon as feasible to ensure that the corneal epithelium is intact. If not, prophylactic antibiotic drops or ointment should be administered to protect the cornea from the pathogens, specifically gram-negative bacteria, that are endemic in most burns units. As the edema subsides, and the eyelids heal, the contracting forces lead to ectropion and corneal exposure. Ectropion may be intrinsic or extrinsic or a combination of both mechanisms. Extrinsic ectropion is caused by the contracting forces of adjacent, burnt facial areas (Fig. 6.47). Intrinsic ectropion results from

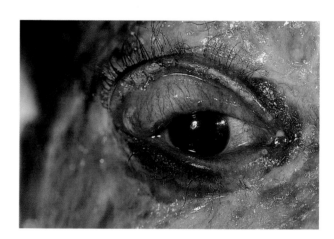

**Figure 6.49** *Ectropion of the upper eyelid caused by a gasoline (petrol) burn.*

contracture of the thin eyelid skin compounded by its close relationship to the underlying pretarsal orbicularis (Fig. 6.48). This distinction is important clinically. Treatment of an extrinsic ectropion requires release or replacement of the adjacent skin, whereas treatment of the intrinsic ectropion requires replacement of the damaged eyelid skin.

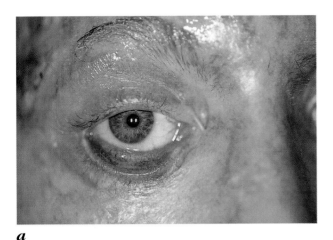

*a*

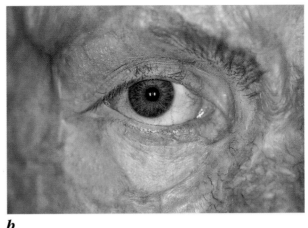

*b*

**Figure 6.50** *Cicatrical, intrinsic ectropion of the lower eyelid (a), treated with full-thickness supraclavicular skin graft and tarsal strip horizontal tightening of the lower eyelid (b).*

Ectropion can involve the upper (Fig. 6.49) or the lower eyelids (Fig. 6.48). Even in full-thickness eyelid burns the deep structures (levator, tarsus and conjunctiva) are usually spared. Treatment consists of release of the contracting forces and full-thickness skin grafting.

An incision is made 1–2 mm below the lash line of the lower eyelid extending from the punctum to the lateral canthus and beyond if necessary. Traction sutures are placed through the eyelid margin and it is placed on upward stretch. The contracture is released with sharp dissection. Complete release is evident when the punctum and the inner lamella of the eyelid lie in apposition to the globe. A Telfa template is cut to the crescent-shaped pattern evident below the eyelid. With the lid on upward stretch, this is approximately 25% larger than actually needed. The size of graft necessary to fill the defect is always surprisingly large. A supraclavicular donor site is necessary to obtain a sufficiently large graft. One should not expect to be able to fill these defects with retroauricular skin. There is simply not enough available. The donor graft is outlined on the supraclavicular site and incised with a blade and dissected free from the underlying tissue with sharp scissors. It is important to thin the graft by excising the excessive subcutaneous tissue. The thinned graft is then sutured into position using alternating 6-0 silk and 6-0 mild chromic suture. The ends of the silk suture are left long and used to fix the Telfa bolster to the wound at the conclusion of the procedure. Medial and lateral tarsorrhaphies may be used to help stabilize the lid and keep it on upward stretch. Repeated skin grafts, Z-plasties and scar revisions are often necessary. The desired result is protection of the eye and the best cosmetic and functional result possible (Fig. 6.50).

Whereas the lower eyelid needs stability, best achieved with a full-thickness skin graft, the upper lid needs mobility. This is best achieved with a very thin full-thickness or partial-thickness skin graft. Grossly ectropic upper eyelids (Fig. 6.49) may require very large skin grafts, and the results are not as good as with lower lid reconstruction. Patients with severe eyelid burns may require multiple reconstructive surgical procedures to protect their eyes and improve their appearance and function (Fig. 6.50).

## SECONDARY REPAIR OF TRAUMATIZED EYELIDS

The eyelids may be damaged by faulty or inexpert primary repair, by cicatrizing changes that cause contracture of the eyelids in spite of seemingly adequate primary repair (Fig. 6.7) and adherence of the eyelids to underlying bone grafts and plates

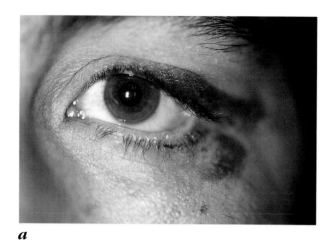

*a*

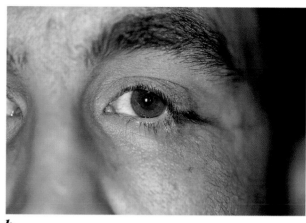

*b*

**Figure 6.51** *Retraction and adherence of the lower eyelid to the orbital rim after reconstructive orbital surgery and multiple attempts at eyelid reconstruction (a). Appearance of lower eyelid after reconstruction with a temporalis-periosteal flap and ear cartilage graft (b).*

placed during orbital reconstructive procedures.[14] These eyelid malpositions may sometimes be easily repaired, as in excising and resuturing a notched eyelid (Fig. 6.31), or may tax the ingenuity of the most experienced oculoplastic surgeon, for example, in repairing an eyelid adherent to the orbital rim (Fig. 6.51).

A lower eyelid notch may be excised primarily and the eyelid resutured as in the primary repair of an eyelid laceration. A double-armed 4-0 silk suture is placed through the notch and the lid put on upward stretch. The notch is excised in a pentagonal fashion (Fig. 6.8) and the resultant defect primarily repaired as described above.

Upper eyelid notches (Fig. 6.31) are more symptomatic, resulting in incomplete closure of the eyelids and corneal exposure. It should be remembered that, when excising a notch from the upper eyelid, the parallel sides of the pentagonal incision must extend the entire vertical height of the tarsus to prevent unsightly and dysfunctional notching, and sutures must not penetrate the conjunctival surface and rub against the cornea (Fig. 6.30).

After reconstructive orbital surgery the lower eyelids may become adherent to the orbital rim and retract from the globe (Fig. 6.51). This is caused by adherence and scarring of the inner lamella of the eyelid to the exposed orbital rim, bone grafts or plates. Repair may entail simply lysing the scars,

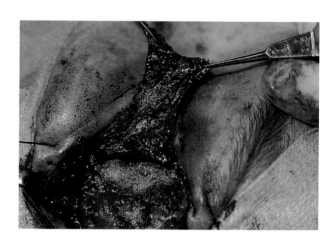

**Figure 6.52** *A vascularized flap of periosteum and temporalis muscle can be mobilized from the lateral orbital wall and is an excellent source of vascular tissue for eyelid reconstruction.*

recessing the conjunctiva and eyelid retractors, and placing the eyelid on upward stretch. Some retracted lids are refractory to standard techniques and may require a bit of ingenuity by the surgeon to resolve the problem. Spacing grafts such as hard palate and ear cartilage may be necessary to elongate the eyelids vertically and obviate the eyelid retraction. These are

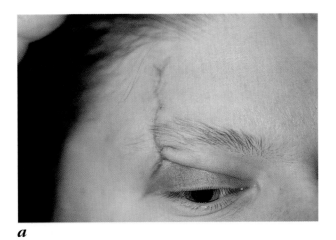

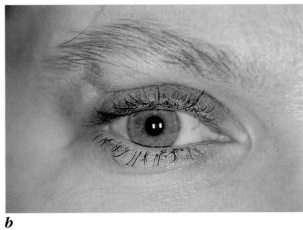

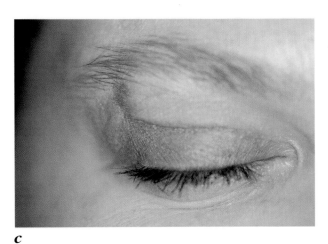

**Figure 6.53** *Retraction and scarring of the upper eyelid (a). Appearance after reconstruction with small Z-plasties and free skin grafts from the opposite eyelid ((b), (c)).*

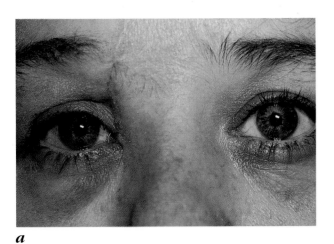

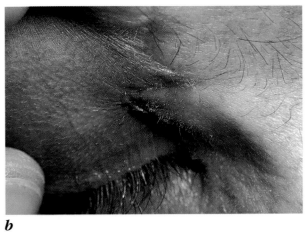

**Figure 6.54** *Webbing of the upper eyelid medial canthal junction.*

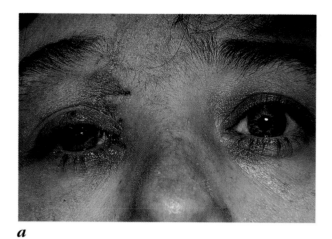

*a*

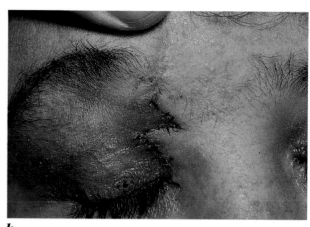

*b*

**Figure 6.55** *Resolution of webbing after a small Z-plasty.*

easily obtained from their respective donor sites. More severe eyelid retraction may be refractory to these relatively simple methods of repair and require more ingenious solutions. A useful alternative is to mobilize a vascular temporalis fascia-periosteal flap from the lateral orbital wall (Fig. 6.52).[15] This flap is vascularized from the inner orbital zygomatico-temporal vessels and is an excellent source of vascularized tissue for eyelid reconstruction.

Retraction and scarring of the upper eyelid can be both unsightly and dysfunctional (Fig. 6.53). This may be repaired by a combination of Z-plasties or free skin grafts from the ipsilateral or the contralateral upper eyelid (Fig. 6.53 (b) and (c)).

Webbing of the medial canthus (Fig. 6.54) may be repaired in a similar fashion with Z-plasties combined with skin grafting as necessary (Fig. 6.55).

## REFERENCES

1  Tenzel RR, Stewart WB. Eyelid reconstruction by a semi-circular flap technique. *Trans Am Soc Ophth & Oto* 1978; **85**: 1164–9.

2  Hughes WH. Total lower eyelid reconstruction. *Trans Am Ophth Soc* 1976; **74**: 321–9.

3  Anderson RL, Gordy DD. The tarsal strip procedure. *Arch Ophthalmol* 1979; **97**: 2192–6.

4  Jordan DR, Anderson RL. The lateral tarsal strip revisited: the enhanced tarsal strip. *Arch Ophthalmol* 1989; **107**: 604–6.

5  Hurwitz JJ. *Lacrimal Surgery.* Philadelphia: Raven-Lippincott, 1996.

6  Reifler DM. Diagnostic and surgical techniques. Management of canalicular laceration. *Surv Ophthalmol* 1991; **36**: 113.

7  Smith B, Petrelli R. Surgical repair of prolapsed lacrimal glands. *Arch Ophthalmol* 1978; **96**: 113–14.

8  Cutler N, Beard C. A method for partial and total upper eyelid reconstruction. *Am J Ophthalmol* 1955; **39**: 1–7.

9  Spinelli HM, Sherman JE et al. Human bites of the eyelid. *Pl Reconst Surg* 1986; **78**: 610.

10  Gonnering RS. Ocular adnexal injury and complications in orbital dig bites. *Ophth Pl Recons Surg* 1987; **3**: 231.

11  Hurwitz JJ, Kratzky V. Dog and human bites of the eyelid respond with retreived autogenous tissue. *Can J Ophthalmol* 1991; **26**: 334–7.

12  Frank DH, Wachtel T, Frank HA. The early treatment and reconstruction of eyelid burns. *J Trauma* 1983; **23**: 874–7.

13  Guy RT et al. Three years experience in a regional burn center with burns of the eyelids. *Ophth Surg* 1982; **13**: 576.

14  Soll DB. Treatment of late traumatic eyelid problems. *Trans Amer Acad Ophth Oto* 1976; **81**: 560.

15  Spoor TC, Ramocki JM, Cowden JC. A periosteal-temporalis flap for repairing impending ocular perforations. *Am J Ophthalmol* 1989; **108**: 704–9.

# *Chapter 7* **Neuro-ophthalmologic manifestations of cranial and ocular trauma**

Neuro-ophthalmologic manifestations of cranio-orbital trauma may be obvious or subtle. Blind is not subtle. Patients with traumatic optic neuropathies and visual loss are aware of this shortly after regaining consciousness. Diagnosis and management are discussed extensively in the chapter on traumatic optic neuropathies.[1]

Little is written about more subtle traumatic optic neuropathies. These patients often travel from doctor to doctor and lawyer to lawyer looking for a diagnosis or compensation for their visual loss. All too often it remains undiagnosed and untreated. The following case is illustrative.

A 40-year-old truck driver struck the back of his head while unloading his truck. He noticed immediate loss of his superior visual field to the extent that he was uncomfortable driving home. He was evaluated by the company physician and told that there was nothing wrong with his vision. He saw several ophthalmologists without obtaining a diagnosis. Visual acuity was 20/20 in each eye. There was no relative afferent pupillary defect, but light-near dissociation of the pupils was evident. Visual fields demonstrated very reproducible, incongruous superior altitudinal scotomas (Fig. 7.1) compatible with the patient's complaints. Fundus examination was initially normal, as was neuroimaging. Repeat visual fields were very reproducible, and subsequent fundus examination demonstrated sector optic atrophy compatible with the reproducible visual field defects (Fig. 7.2).

The case illustrates several important concepts to consider when treating patients with craniocervical injuries and ocular complaints. First, the patient has

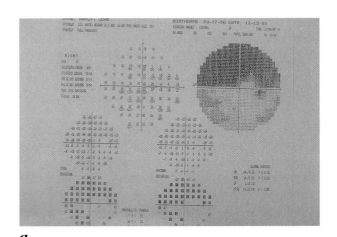
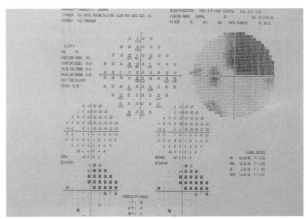

*a*  *b*

**Figure 7.1** *Visual fields demonstrating incongruous altitudinal defects.*

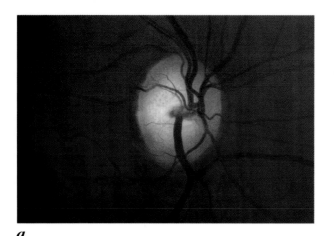
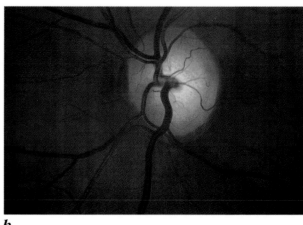

*a*                                              *b*

**Figure 7.2** *Sector optic atrophy compatible with visual field defects.*

a problem until proven otherwise. Just because the physician is not astute enough to recognize and diagnose the problem does not negate its presence. It is very easy to denigrate a patient's complaints, especially when they follow a compensation-type injury. It is important to realize that the patient has a problem until proven otherwise. He/she is innocent until proven guilty.

Loss of visual acuity or field after a craniocervical injury may result from an injury to the optic nerves, chiasm or occipital cortex. Automated perimetry should yield appropriate and reproducible results. Pupillary examination should enable the examiner to differentiate between optic nerve or chiasmal injury and occipital cortex injury. Patients with optic nerve or chiasmal injuries will have pupillary abnormalities. If an obvious relative afferent pupillary defect is not present, light-near dissociation of the pupils should be sought, signifying bilateral optic nerve or chiasmal injury as in the previously described case.

Traumatic optic nerve injuries may be obvious (Fig. 7.3) or very subtle, only evident after a careful history and neuro-ophthalmologic examination. The author suspects injury to the optic nerve in any patient who has had significant head trauma. A careful pupillary examination, formal visual fields and specific questions concerning light and color desaturation should precede examination of the optic nerve looking for evidence of subtle optic atrophy.

## CHIASMAL TRAUMA

Bilateral optic nerve injuries (Fig. 7.3) may be confused with traumatic injuries to the optic chiasm. These injuries are uncommon, but patients present with variations upon the theme of bitemporal hemianopia with or without diabetes insipidus panhypopituitarism, traumatic carotid aneurysms, carotid cavernous fistulae and cerebrospinal fluids (CSF) leaks.[2,3] Bilateral pupillary dysfunction—light-near dissociation—is the hallmark of bilateral optic nerve or chiasmal injury. An obvious relative afferent pupillary defect may not be present in patients with chiasmal dysfunction; however, light-near dissociation will always be present if sought. The site of injury is often difficult to detect neuroradiologically. Magnetic resonance imaging (MRI) is most accurate for delineating the etiology of chiasmal trauma.[4] Diagnosis is predicated upon an initially normal fundus examination. Optic atrophy will eventually ensue. Bilateral choroidal tears, or unilateral traumatic optic neuropathy and a contralateral choroidal tear may mimic a chiasmal syndrome.

The chiasm may be damaged by transection, contusion, hemorrhage, and inferior herniation of the rectus gyrus.[4] Chiasmal trauma should be suspected in patients with frontal injuries and basilar skull fractures.[5] It needs to be differentiated from bilateral

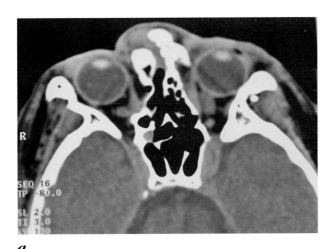

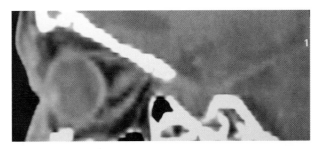

*b*

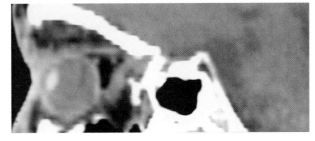

*a*

**Figure 7.3** *CT scans (axial (a)) and sagittal ((b) and (c)) demonstrating bilateral transection of the optic nerves in a patient bilaterally blind after severe midface trauma.*

*c*

optic nerve injury. Delayed, progressive bilateral visual loss may occur days after frontal head trauma due to intrachiasmal hemorrhage.[6] MRI will demonstrate chiasmal hemorrhage and edema. Chiasmal injury is more prone to be accompanied by other neurologic deficits. Associated epistaxis should alert the clinician to a concomitant carotid artery injury. Patients with associated CSF leaks are at high risk for developing meningitis. These patients are at high risk for a catastrophic event and require multidisciplinary intervention sooner rather than later.

Treatment for traumatic chiasmal injuries entails accurate diagnosis and treatment of concomitant endocrinologic and neurologic dysfunction. MRI greatly facilitates the diagnosis and etiology of post-traumatic chiasmal visual dysfunction. A course of megadose corticosteroids, as given for traumatic optic neuropathies, might help and probably will not hurt the patient.

## OCCIPITAL TRAUMA

If pupillary reactions are normal after careful examination (preferably on several occasions by several examiners), occipital cortex injury as the etiology of the visual dysfunction should be considered. These

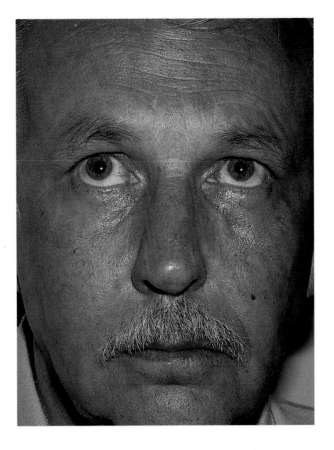

**Figure 7.4** *Patient awakening from cardiac bypass surgery with bilateral visual loss.*

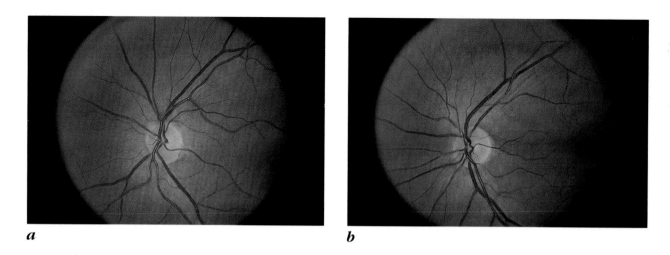

*a*        *b*

**Figure 7.5** *Fundus examination was normal. Pupillary examination was normal.*

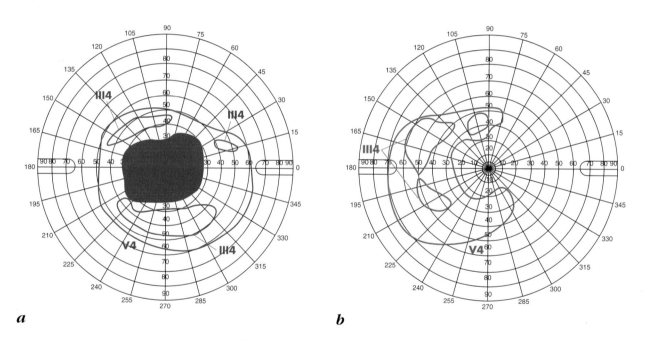

*a*        *b*

**Figure 7.6** *Visual fields demonstrate large bilateral central scotomas.*

patients will have very reproducible, very congruent visual field defects accompanied by a normal ocular and pupillary examination.

There are two types of occipital cortex injuries—hypoperfusion and infarction, or direct trauma to the occipital lobe. Patients experiencing massive blood loss or significant hypotension may suffer a watershed-type infarction of the occipital cortex. These patients present with bilateral central visual loss (Figs 7.4–7.7). Patients awake after injury complaining of bilateral visual loss. Their ocular examination is normal (Fig. 7.5). Their visual fields demonstrate a significant bilateral deficit (Fig. 7.6) which may improve significantly with time (Fig. 7.7). The occipital tip, serving macular vision, is

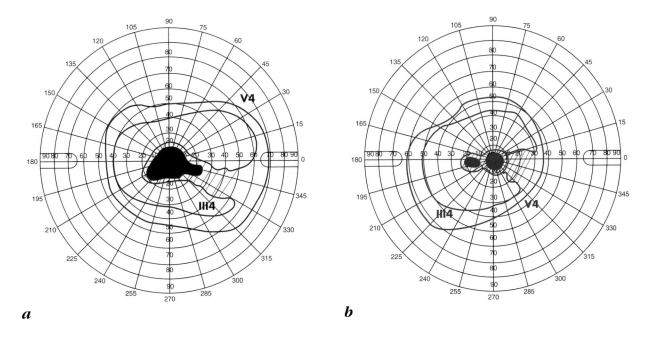

**Figure 7.7** *Partial resolution of central scotomas still results in very significant visual dysfunction.*

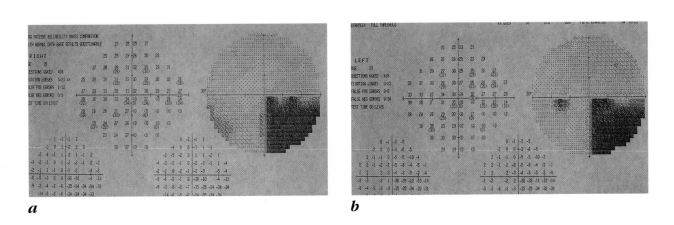

**Figure 7.8** *Very homonymous inferior quadrantanopia due to occipital lobe injury.*

most susceptible to this watershed-type infarction which often results in bilateral central visual loss.

Injury to the occipital cortex results in very homonymous visual field defects (Fig. 7.8) that spare central fixation. These patients have normal visual acuity but have a visual field defect that may be documented on automated perimetry. Neuroimaging studies may initially fail to demonstrate occipital injury or infarction, but eventually there will be a defect present that correlates with the visual field defect. MR scanning is very useful in localizing the defective area of occipital cortex (Figs 7.9 and 7.10).

Rarely, occipital injuries may be combined with elevated intracranial pressure and optic nerve

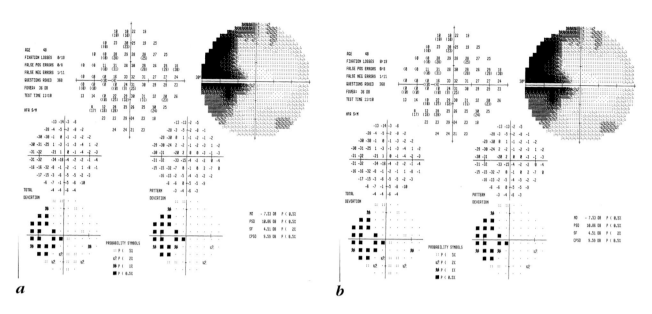

**Figure 7.9** *Very homonymous hemianopias secondary to occipital lobe infarction.*

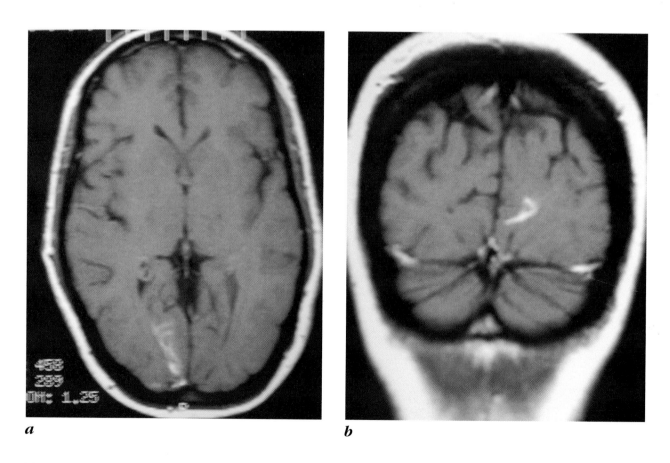

**Figure 7.10** *MR scan demonstrating occipital lobe infarction presenting as very homonymous hemianopias in Fig. 7.9 ((a) axial, (b) coronal).*

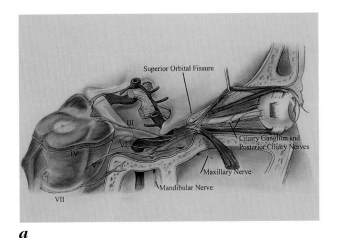

*a*

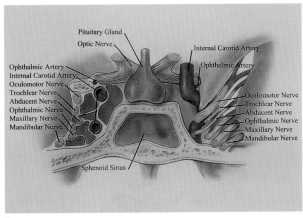

*b*

**Figure 7.11** *The oculomotor nerves passing from the brainstem, through the cavernous sinus and into the orbit (a). Relationship of cranial nerves in the cavernous sinus (b).*

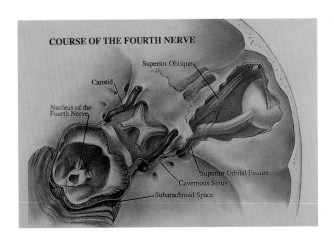

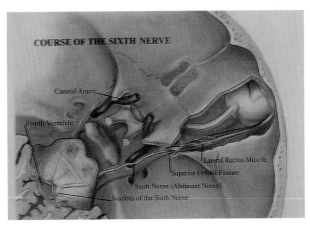

**Figure 7.12** *The intracranial course of the fourth cranial nerve.*

**Figure 7.13** *The intracranial course of the sixth cranial nerve.*

dysfunction. These patients need to have their untreatable occipital lobe injury differentiated from their potentially treatable optic neuropathy. Awareness and proper examination of the pupils is the key to diagnosis, and appropriate treatment is predicated upon accurate diagnosis.

Children may develop transient cortical blindness after significant or sometimes even trivial occipital or frontal trauma.[7] Onset of blindness may be immediate or occur 10–15 minutes after injury. These children cannot fixate, follow a light, respond to a visual threat, or follow their eyes in a mirror. Pupillary reactions are normal; the neuro-ophthalmic examination is normal excepting absent optokinetic responses. Blindness lasts minutes to hours, and the prognosis for recovery is usually excellent.

Injuries to the temporal and parietal lobes may also cause a visual field defect. Temporal lobe injury may cause a superior quadrantanopia (pie in the sky) field defect. If complete, it is impossible to distinguish

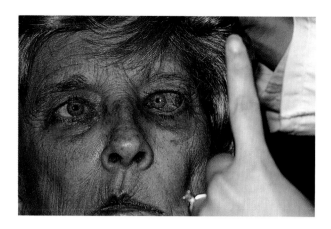

**Figure 7.14** *Patient with a sixth and seventh cranial nerve palsy secondary to a basilar skull fracture.*

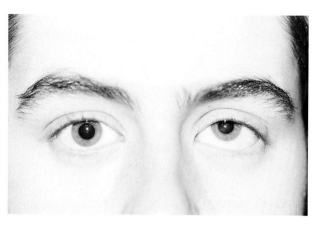

**Figure 7.15** *Patient with a large left hypertropia (LHT) after head injury.*

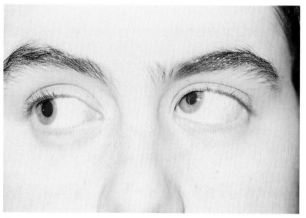

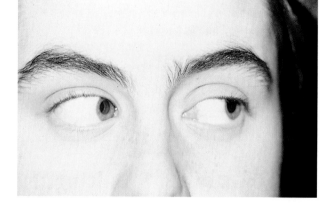

*a*

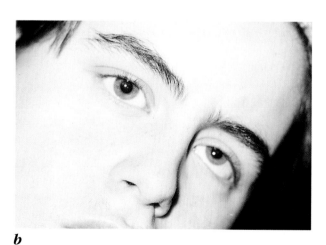

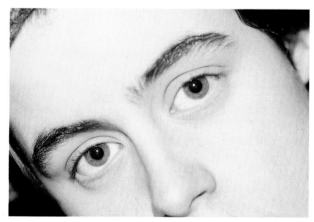

*b*

**Figure 7.16** *Three-step test. Patient with an LHT due to a left superior oblique palsy. The LHT increases in right gaze and decreases in left gaze (a). LHT increases with left head tilt and decreases in right head tilt (b).*

from an occipital lobe defect. If incomplete, temporal lobe defects tend to be more incongruous than the occipital lobe defects. Parietal lobe injuries may result in an inferior quadrantanopia. Both temporal and parietal lobe visual field defects are rarely isolated sequelae of neurologic trauma. These may also be seen as sequelae to neurosurgical intervention in a traumatized brain.

## EXTRAOCULAR MOTILITY DYSFUNCTION

Diplopia is a common complaint in patients suffering cranio-orbital trauma.[8,9] The three oculomotor nerves are quite susceptible to injury as they course from the brainstem to and through the cavernous sinus (Figs 7.11 (a) and (b)). The fourth and sixth cranial nerves are most susceptible to injury (Figs 7.12 and 7.13). The fourth nerve, as it exits the dorsal brainstem, is susceptible to shearing forces caused by closed head or craniocervical injuries (Fig. 7.12). The sixth nerve has a long course along the base of the skull (Fig. 7.13). It is susceptible to the same mechanisms of injury as the fourth nerve and may also be injured with or without an accompanying facial nerve palsy by base of the skull fractures (Fig. 7.14).

The cause of a patient's diplopia may be very obvious if a single cranial nerve is injured. Isolated fourth- and sixth-nerve palsies are common and easily differentiated. Trauma causes approximately 32% of fourth-nerve palsies.[10] The patient with a

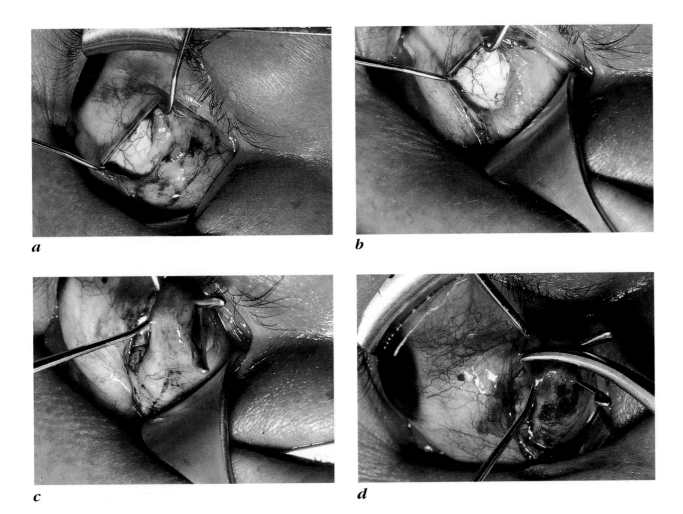

*a.*

*b*

*c*

*d*

**Figure 7.17** *Inferior oblique recession: the lateral and inferior recti are isolated with muscle hooks and retracted (a). As the recti are retracted, the conjunctiva is retracted exposing the inferior oblique (b). Under direct visualization the inferior oblique is completely isolated with two muscle hooks (c). The isolated muscle is clamped, cauterized and cut under direct visualization (d).*

fourth-nerve palsy (Fig. 7.15) complains of vertical diplopia and will have a positive three-step test (Fig. 7.16). This diagnosis should be easily made in the office, but may be harder at the bedside, especially if the patient is tested in the supine position. The three-step test cannot be performed in the supine position for the ocular torsion response is based upon the otolith's response to gravity. The vertical deviation is also often more obvious when the patient is erect.

As with other cranial nerve palsies, treatment is observation for a least 6 months in hopes of spontaneous recovery. Press-on Fresnel prisms (3M Healthcare, St Paul, MN) may help obviate the diplopia while awaiting spontaneous resolution. After 6 months, an overacting inferior oblique may be recessed or myotomized; an underacting but functioning superior oblique may be tucked. In patients with long-standing superior oblique paresis, a spread of comitance may have occurred; recession of the contralateral inferior oblique may be a useful procedure to obviate the diplopia. The author routinely weakens overacting inferior oblique muscles and rarely strengthens underacting superior oblique muscles. Others prefer superior oblique tucking procedures. Inferior oblique weakening can be quickly and easily performed under local anesthesia; in patients with overacting inferior obliques it is quite helpful in obviating diplopia.

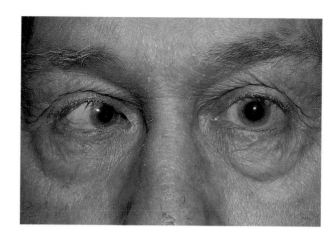

**Figure 7.18** *Patient with a left six-nerve palsy.*

The key to successful inferior oblique surgery is isolation of the muscle under direct visualization. An oblique incision is made in the inferior temporal quadrant of the eye through conjunctiva and Tenon's capsule. The inferior rectus and the lateral rectus are isolated with muscle hooks (Fig. 7.17(a)) and retracted. A DesMarres retractor is used to retract the conjunctiva

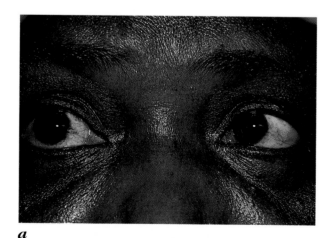

*a*

**Figure 7.19** *Patient with a right six-nerve palsy (a) adapts a compensatory left face turn to look away from the paretic muscle and avoid diplopia.*

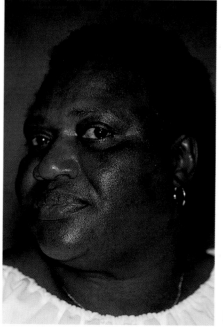

*b*

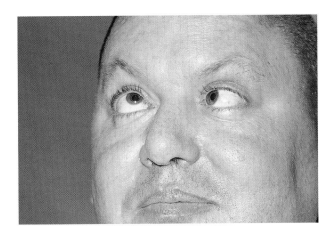

**Figure 7.20** *Bilateral six-nerve palsy caused by a severe head injury.*

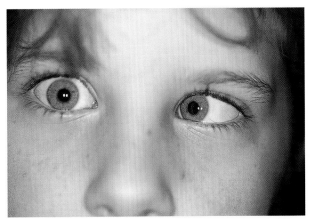

*a*

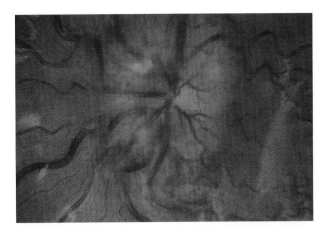

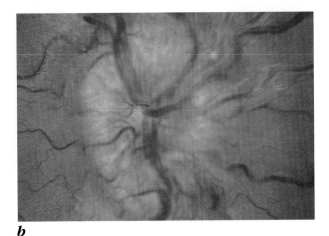

*b*

**Figure 7.21** *Right six-nerve palsy secondary to elevated intracranial pressure (a). Fundus examination demonstrates florid papilledema (b).*

and expose the inferior oblique under direct visualization (Fig. 7.17(b)). The exposed inferior oblique is isolated with muscle hooks (Fig. 7.17(c)), clamped, cauterized and transected (Fig. 7.17(d)). The transected muscle may then be myotomized or recessed. The author's practice is to cut off a piece of the muscle and suture it into its capsule so that it cannot inadvertently advance towards its original position. Recession of the muscle to the lateral border of the inferior rectus takes longer and accomplishes the same goal.

If the surgeon elects to recess the contralateral inferior rectus, 1 mm of recession will correct approximately 3 prism diopters of hypotropia. The author only recesses the contralateral inferior rectus in patients who have a long-standing superior oblique palsy with spread of comitance or in patients whose deviation was not adequately corrected after an inferior oblique weakening procedure.

Trauma causes approximately 17% of sixth-nerve palsies.[10] A patient with a sixth-nerve paresis (Fig. 7.18) complains of horizontal diplopia, increasing in the field of action of the involved muscle-abduction of the eye, and may adapt a compensatory head position, turning away from the involved muscle (Fig. 7.19). Bilateral sixth-nerve palsies are quite obvious (Fig. 7.20) and very disconcerting to the patient. They are usually the result of very significant craniocervical trauma. A unilateral or bilateral sixth-nerve palsy may also result from elevated intracranial pressure. Treatment is normalization of intracranial pressure (Fig. 7.21). Sixth-nerve palsies may be accompanied by an ipsilateral seventh-nerve palsy due to basilar

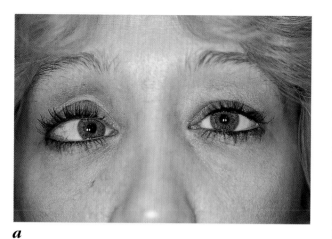 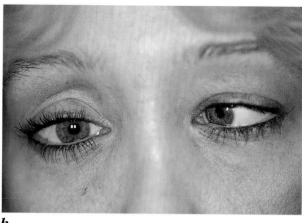

**Figure 7.22** *Patient with a left six-nerve palsy in primary gaze (a) and in left gaze (b).*

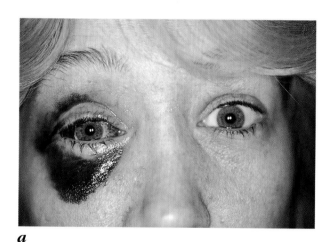 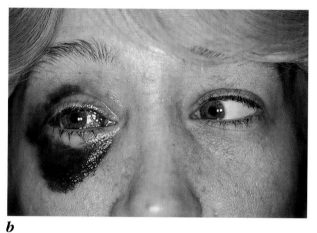

**Figure 7.23** *Patient after Hummelsheim transposition procedure now straight in primary gaze (a) with some abduction (b).*

skull fractures (Fig. 7.14). These patients may have difficulty closing their eyes and develop an exposure keratopathy. The cornea needs to be protected while awaiting resolution of the cranial nerve palsies.

Traditional treatment is observation for 6 months followed by eye muscle surgery. If partial function has returned, diplopia may be obviated by a recession of the medial rectus and resection of the lateral rectus. If no sixth-nerve function returns, a transposi-

tion procedure may be performed. The medial rectus is recessed maximally (6 mm) and the lateral halves of the superior and inferior recti are transposed to the insertion of the lateral rectus. This straightens the eye in primary gaze and allows some abduction (Fig. 7.22 and 7.23).

Acute sixth-nerve palsies may also be treated by injection of Oculinum (Botox, Allergan, Irvine, CA) into the ipsilateral medial rectus muscle.

Pharmacologic paralysis of the medial rectus prevents contracture from working unopposed against a paretic lateral rectus and may offer a better prognosis for recovery of binocular vision without surgery. This treatment, although promising, has neither withstood the test of time nor undergone a randomized clinical trial.

## THIRD-NERVE PALSY

Fortunately, third-nerve palsies are not as common a sequela of head injury as fourth- and sixth-nerve palsies. Trauma accounts for 16% of third-nerve palsies.[10] The third nerve subserves multiple extraocular muscles, the levator and accommodation. Injury is potentially much more disabling and far less treatable than injury to the other oculomotor nerves which enervate just one extraocular muscle.

As with other post-traumatic oculomotor nerve palsies, treatment is initially observation and hope for spontaneous recovery of some or all of the motility function. If recovery occurs it usually happens within 3–6 months. Total or partial recovery of third-nerve function may be accompanied by aberrant regeneration with an interesting synkinesis between extraocular movements and eyelid or pupillary function (Fig. 7.24).

Partial resolution of third-nerve function may allow surgical correction of the motility defect. The horizontal component may totally or partially resolve, leaving a large vertical deviation (Fig. 7.25), or the vertical component may resolve, leaving a large horizontal deviation (Fig. 7.26). Often the resolution is partial. These are very difficult problems to correct surgically; however, at least if some function recovers, patients have a chance of obtaining binocular visual function in some fields of gaze. There is no good treatment for a total third-nerve palsy that fails to recover any function.

## MULTIPLE CRANIAL NERVE PALSIES

Multiple cranial nerve palsies (Fig. 7.27) are usually due to more severe head trauma with fractures of the sphenoid, petrous temporal or orbital bones. Head trauma causes approximately 20% of single and multiple cranial nerve palsies.[10] Paresis of any combination of cranial nerves III, IV and VI may occur. Treatment entails observation for spontaneous resolution or at least improvement and then attempts at corrective extraocular muscle surgery. Recovery of function occurs in approximately 40% of traumatic cranial nerve palsies whether they are isolated or multiple.[8,10]

Carotid-cavernous fistulas may occur after head injury and present with any combination of cranial nerve palsies (Fig. 7.28). The sixth nerve is the most frequently affected because it lies free in the cavernous sinus (Fig. 7.11(b)). The third and fourth cranial nerves lie in the dural walls of the cavernous sinus and are not as frequently involved. Occasionally all cranial nerves are affected, and these patients present with a frozen globe (Fig. 7.28). This diagnosis is rarely subtle.

## CONCOMITANT DEVIATIONS

Concomitant exo- and esodeviations may occur after head trauma. Esotropia secondary to a partially resolved sixth-nerve palsy may result in a concomitant deviation of 25 prism diopters – a blind spot syndrome. The patient fixates the deviated image on the optic nerve to avoid diplopia. Eye muscle surgery often resolves the esodeviations (Fig. 7.29) resulting in straight eyes and fusion. Patients with post-traumatic exodeviations do not fare as well. Often these patients do not have resolution of the objective angle of deviation or their diplopia in spite of seemingly adequate surgery.[9] There is no good explanation as to why these patients do not improve, but it is disconcerting to both patient and physician. Awareness of the poor surgical prognosis prior to surgery keeps patient expectations at a reasonable level.

## CONVERGENCE ACCOMMODATIVE INSUFFICIENCY

Problems with accommodation and/or convergence are common sequelae of head injury, occurring in 36% of patients recovering from head trauma.[9] These patients may present with isolated defective accommodation, convergence or both. It may resolve spontaneously (approximately 50%) or be refractory to treat-

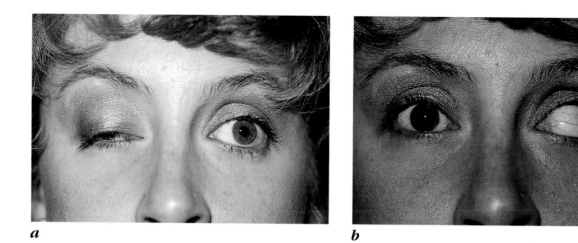

*a*                                    *b*

**Figure 7.24** *Patient with ptosis secondary to a third-nerve palsy (a). Resolution of ptosis with attempted adduction of the right eye due to aberrant regeneration (b).*

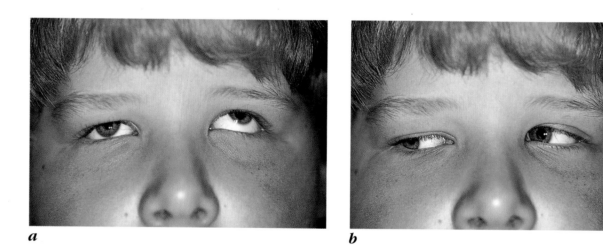

*a*                                    *b*

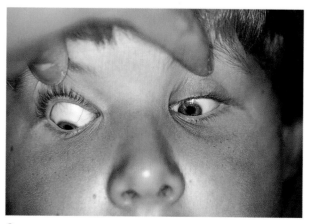

**Figure 7.25** *Patient with partial resolution of a third-nerve palsy with a large left hypertropia (a). Almost full restoration of adduction (b) with residual defective depression of the left eye (c).*

*c*

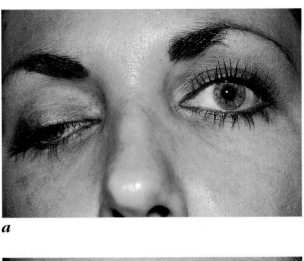

*a*

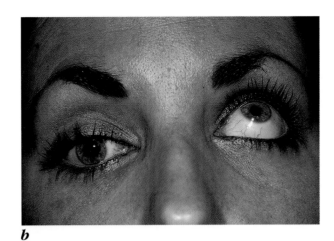

*b*

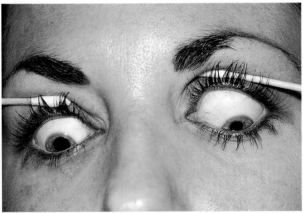

*c*

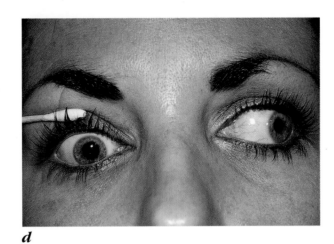

*d*

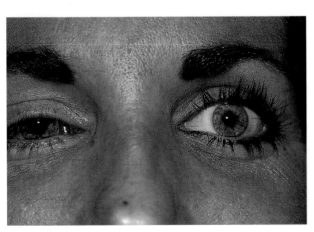

*e*

**Figure 7.26** *Partially resolved third-nerve palsy with ptosis and a large exotropia (a). Elevation (b) and adduction are severely limited (c). Depression of the right eye has normalized (d). Eyes are straight after horizontal muscle surgery (e). Ptosis was not repaired due to defective elevation of the eye (b).*

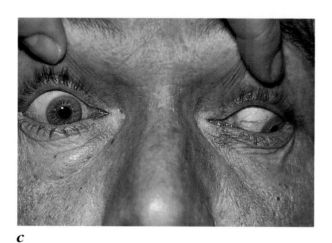

*a*

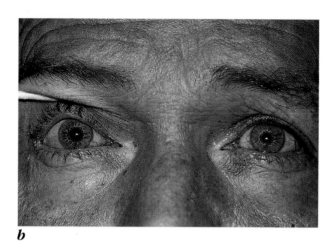

*b*

**Figure 7.27** *Combination third and six cranial nerve palsy secondary to cavernous sinus trauma. Note the ptosis, dilated pupil and adduction defect in the right eye (a–c). Abduction deficit manifestation of the sixth-nerve involvement (d).*

*c*

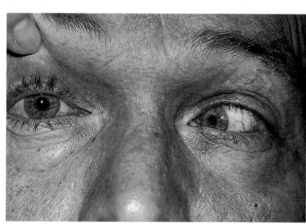

*d*

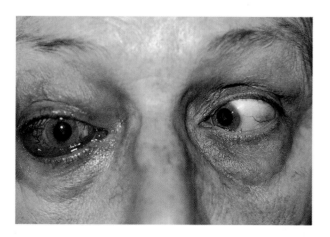

**Figure 7.28** *Patient with a frozen globe secondary to a carotid cavernous fistula. Marked chemosis, arterialization of the conjunctival vessels and a loud bruit made this diagnosis obvious.*

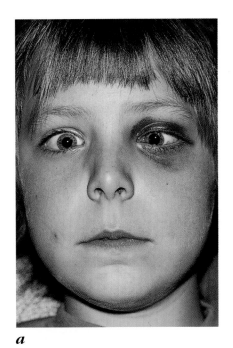

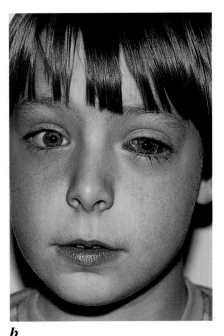

*a*                    *b*

**Figure 7.29** *Partially resolved sixth-nerve palsy (a); eyes straightened by recession of the medial rectus and resection of the lateral rectus 8 months later (b).*

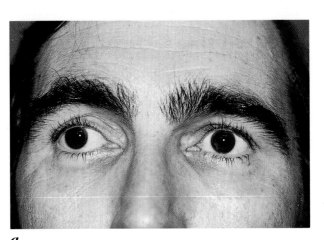

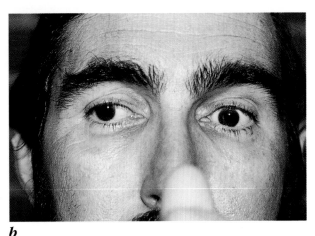

*a*                    *b*

**Figure 7.30** *Exotropia (a) and loss of convergence (b) in a patient with severe convergence insufficiency after closed head injury.*

ment. These patients may present with either loss of accommodation, convergence, or both. The diagnosis may be very obvious, with the patient totally unable to converge his eyes and a manifest exotropia at near (Fig. 7.30). It may also be quite subtle, only evident after listening to the patient's complaints of headache, blurring and diplopia with near effort. Diagnosis is confirmed by noting decreased accommodation and/or convergence amplitudes.

## SPASM OF THE NEAR REFLEX

Pseudomyopia secondary to accommodative spasm and spasm of the near reflex entailing spasm of accommodation (pseudomyopia), convergence, and miosis of the pupils (Fig. 7.31) are also sequelae to head trauma and may very difficult to treat even after an accurate diagnosis has been made. These patients

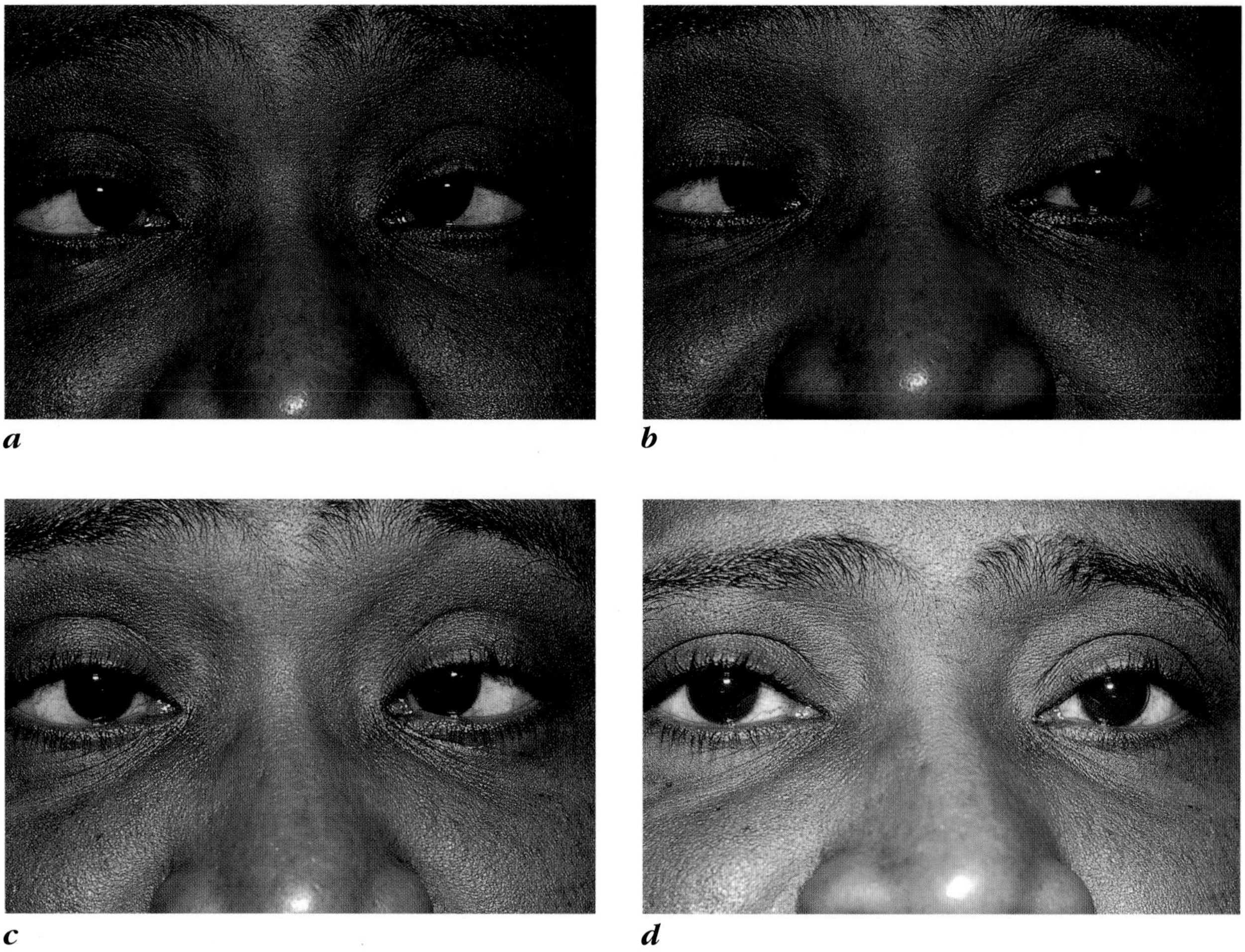

**Figure 7.31** *Spasm of the near reflex mimicking a bilateral sixth-nerve palsy (a–c). Pupil miosis on attempted abduction of either eye and neurologic findings are inconsistent as evidenced by resolution of deviation later in the day (d).*

complain of blurred distance vision and headache. The key to making the diagnosis is recognition of the pseudomyopia—the patient's inability to see clearly in the distance and ability to see normally. Cycloplegic refraction obviates the pseudomyopia and restores distance acuity. The motility deficits are also atypical, do not fit an obvious neurologic pattern, and usually involve defective ocular abduction (Fig. 7.31). Noting that the pupil remains miotic on attempted abduction helps elucidate the diagnosis.

## EVALUATION AND TREATMENT

Patients with head injuries should undergo a neuro-ophthalmologic examination including formal perimetry if their mental status permits. Attention should be directed at detecting subtle optic nerve or occipital field defects and the motility dysfunctions described above. An orthoptic evaluation with formal measurement of accommodation and convergence amplitudes helps detect these common sequelae of head injury. Subsequent treatment may be very difficult for both physician and patient. Obvious cranial nerve palsies are observed for resolution and subsequently operated upon if they fail to resolve totally. Accommodative insufficiency may be treated with an appropriate reading add. Convergence insuf-

ficiency may improve with prism exercises. Spasm of the near reflex and pseudomyopia are much more difficult to treat. Sometimes atropinization with a near add for reading, and sunglasses for resultant photophobia are beneficial. Often, however, it is unsuccessful.

## REFERENCES

1  Sofferman RA. The recovery potential of the optic nerve. *Laryngoscope* 1995; **105**: 1–38.
2  Tang RA, Kramer LA, Schiffman J et al. Chiasmal trauma. Clinical imaging and considerations. *Surv Ophthalmol* 1994; **38**: 381–3.
3  Neetens A. Traumatic chiasmal syndrome. *Neuro-ophthalmology* 1992; **12**: 375–82.
4  Marks AS, Phister SH, Jackson DE, Kolsky MP. Traumatic lesion of the suprasellar region—MR imaging. *Radiology* 1992; **187**: 49–52.
5  Heinz GW, Nunery WR, Grossman CB. Traumatic chiasmal syndrome associated with midline basilar skull fractures. *Am J Ophthalmol* 1994; **117**: 90–6.
6  Crowe NW, Nickles TT, Troost BT, Elster AD. Intrachiasmal hemorrhage: a cause of delayed post-traumatic blindness. *Neurology* 1989; **39**: 863–5.
7  Wong VCN. Cortical blindness in children. A study of etiology and prognosis. *Pediatric Neurology* 1991; **7**: 178–85.
8  Baker RS, Epstein AD. Ocular motor abnormalities from head trauma. *Surv Ophthalmol* 1991; **35**: 245–67.
9  Kowal L. Ophthalmic manifestations of head injury. *Aust N Z J Ophthalmol* 1992; **20**: 35–40.
10  Rush JA, Younge B. Paralysis of cranial nerves III, IV and VI: causes and prognosis in 1000 cases. *Arch Ophthalmol* 1981; **99**: 76–9.

# Chapter 8 Penetrating orbital injuries

When evaluating any patient with a periorbital injury, especially a penetrating injury, it must be remembered that the eye and the structures subserving it are surrounded by the bony orbit. Superior and adjacent to the orbital roof is the anterior cranial fossa, medially the ethmoid sinus, inferiorly the maxillary sinus and deep lies the middle cranial fossa (Figs 8.1–8.3). Awareness of these relationships will help avoid both errors of omission and commission when treating patients with injuries to this region.

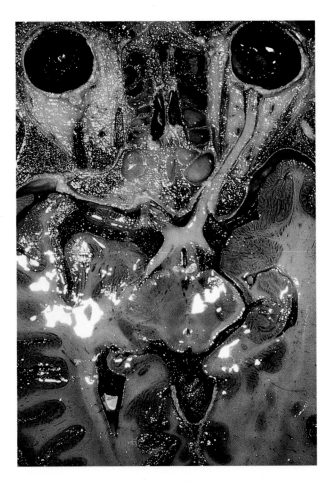

**Figure 8.1** *Axial cadaver section through the mid-orbital plane. The middle cranial fossa lies deep above the orbit, the ethmoid sinus lies medial to the orbit. Note the course of the optic nerve from the back of the eye through the optic canal and intracranially to the optic chiasm.*

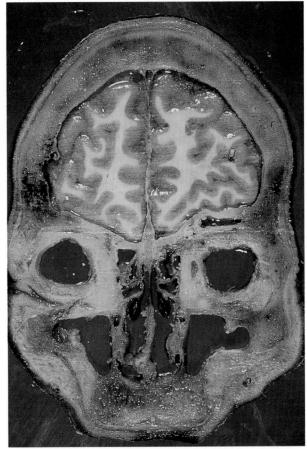

**Figure 8.2** *Coronal cadaver section through the mid-orbit. Note that the orbit is bound superiorly by the anterior cranial fossa, inferiorly by the maxillary sinus and medially by the ethmoid sinus.*

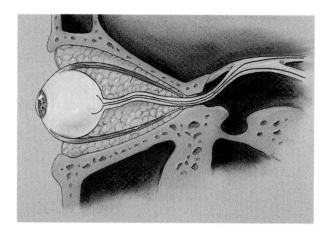

**Figure 8.3** *Diagrammatic sagittal section showing the relationships of the orbit to the brain and sinuses.*

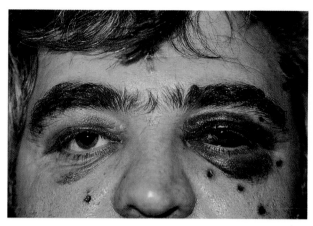

**Figure 8.4** *Pellet wounds to orbit with globe totally spared.*

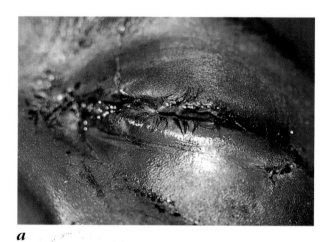

*a*

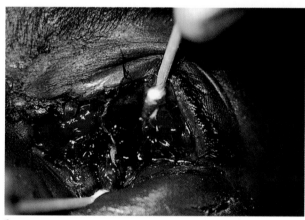

*b*

**Figure 8.5** *Gunshot wound causing total destruction of the eye. This eye was not repairable and was primarily enucleated.*

The major pitfall in managing a patient with a periorbital injury is failure to detect and treat intraocular or intracranial involvement. Any periorbital penetrating injury is an intraocular and/or intracranial injury until proven otherwise. Expect the worst and you will not neglect a potentially treatable injury to the eye or brain. Multiple pellet injuries commonly involve the eye, orbit and brain. The eye may be totally spared or totally destroyed (Figs 8.4–8.6). If the eye is intact, further evaluation should include extraocular motility, and lacrimal excretory and optic nerve functions. If intracranial involvement is present (Fig. 8.6 (d)) the appropriate neurosurgical consultations should be obtained.

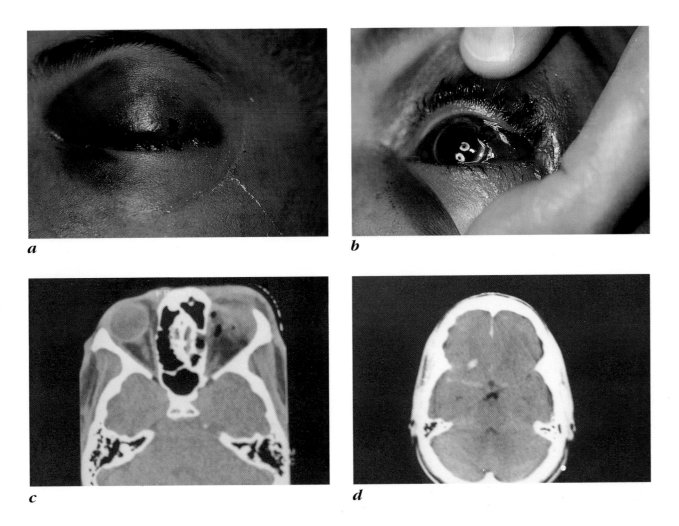

**Figure 8.6** *Periorbital shotgun wound causing a repairable injury to the globe ((a), (b), (c)) as well as intracranial involvement (d).*

Computed tomography remains the most valuable adjunct in investigating penetrating orbital injuries. CT scans can help evaluate the integrity of the globe or the presence of an intraocular foreign body when the media is hazy. It can detect occult intracranial penetration, for example, pneumocephalus (Fig. 8.6 (d)) and can document the type and location of the orbital foreign body. Computed tomography is an integral part of the decision-making process when evaluating penetrating orbital injuries and should be ordered without hesitation.

A penetrating orbital injury may injure the eye in a number of ways, by direct penetration or by concus-sive effect. Visual function may also be affected by penetrating or concussive damage to the optic nerve, extraocular muscles or oculomotor nerves. Chronic compression or infection may affect visual function long after the injury, especially if the injury was occult (Fig. 8.7).

Ocular damage caused by an orbital foreign body depends upon the size, location, composition and ballistics (mass, velocity and fragmentation). Large and slow-moving foreign bodies, for example, knives and sticks, have a tendency to slide along the medial orbital wall, damaging orbital apical structures and causing amaurosis and an orbital apex syndrome

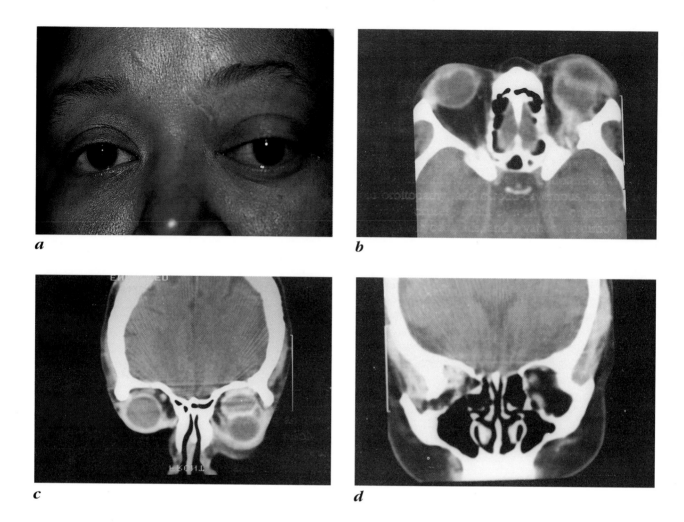

**Figure 8.7** *Orbital abscess appearing many years after occult injury to orbit with a bamboo whip (a). CT scans demonstrate an anterior orbital abscess (b, axial, c, coronal) and retained foreign bodies at the orbital apex (d). Treatment consisted of surgical drainage of the abscess and removal of the wooden foreign bodies.*

(Fig. 8.8). These patients present with ptosis, ophthalmoplegia and amaurosis. Sometimes the optic nerve may be spared. These lucky patients present with ophthalmoplegia, ptosis and normal vision (Figs 8.9 and 8.10). Conventional wisdom states that these changes are permanent; but the author's experience has been that the motility invariably improves regardless of treatment and that the amaurosis may improve with medical or surgical therapy (see Chapter 11).

The patient in Figure 8.8 was assaulted and stabbed in the superomedial orbit. He noted immediate amaurosis and ptosis. An emergency-room consultant documented total ophthalmoplegia and no perception of light. Computed tomography was normal, and the wound was sutured. Four days later he presented for a second opinion. He had total amaurosis and ophthalmoplegia (Fig. 8.8). The pupil was amaurotic, and the fundus was normal (Fig. 8.11). In the spirit of the time, he was treated with a three-day course of megadose corticosteroids (see Chapter 11). His vision promptly improved to 20/100 with a significant residual visual field defect and optic atrophy (Fig. 8.12). The ophthalmoplegia and ptosis resolved within one month (Fig. 8.13).

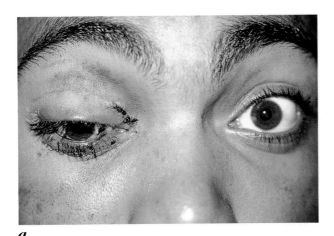

*a*

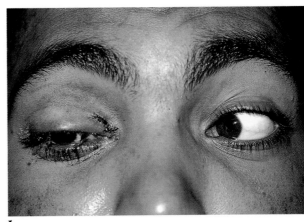

*b*

**Figure 8.8** *Stab wound to medial orbit causing immediate, total blindness and ophthalmoplegia.*

*c*

The patient in Fig. 8.14 had a similar history, except that he was stabbed up the nose with a stiletto and noted immediate blindness and ptosis. Visual acuity of no light perception, an amaurotic pupil, normal fundus and total ophthalmoplegia were documented on initial examination. He was treated with a five-day course of megadose corticosteroids and remained totally blind and ophthalmoplegic on the involved side. He underwent a transethmoidal optic canal decompression. Immediately after surgery, definite light perception was noted; five days later, visual acuity had improved to 20/50 with a peripheral visual field defect (Fig. 8.15). His ophthalmoplegia also resolved.

Both of these patients had 'untreatable' penetrating orbital injuries with total loss of visual function. Both recovered significant visual function and normal extraocular motility. Visual function may have recovered spontaneously; but this is doubtful. Transected optic nerves do not regain function and are untreatable. Obviously there are secondary effects of penetrating injury, most likely hemorrhage and edema, that may be amenable to treatment. It is important to keep an open mind with reference to

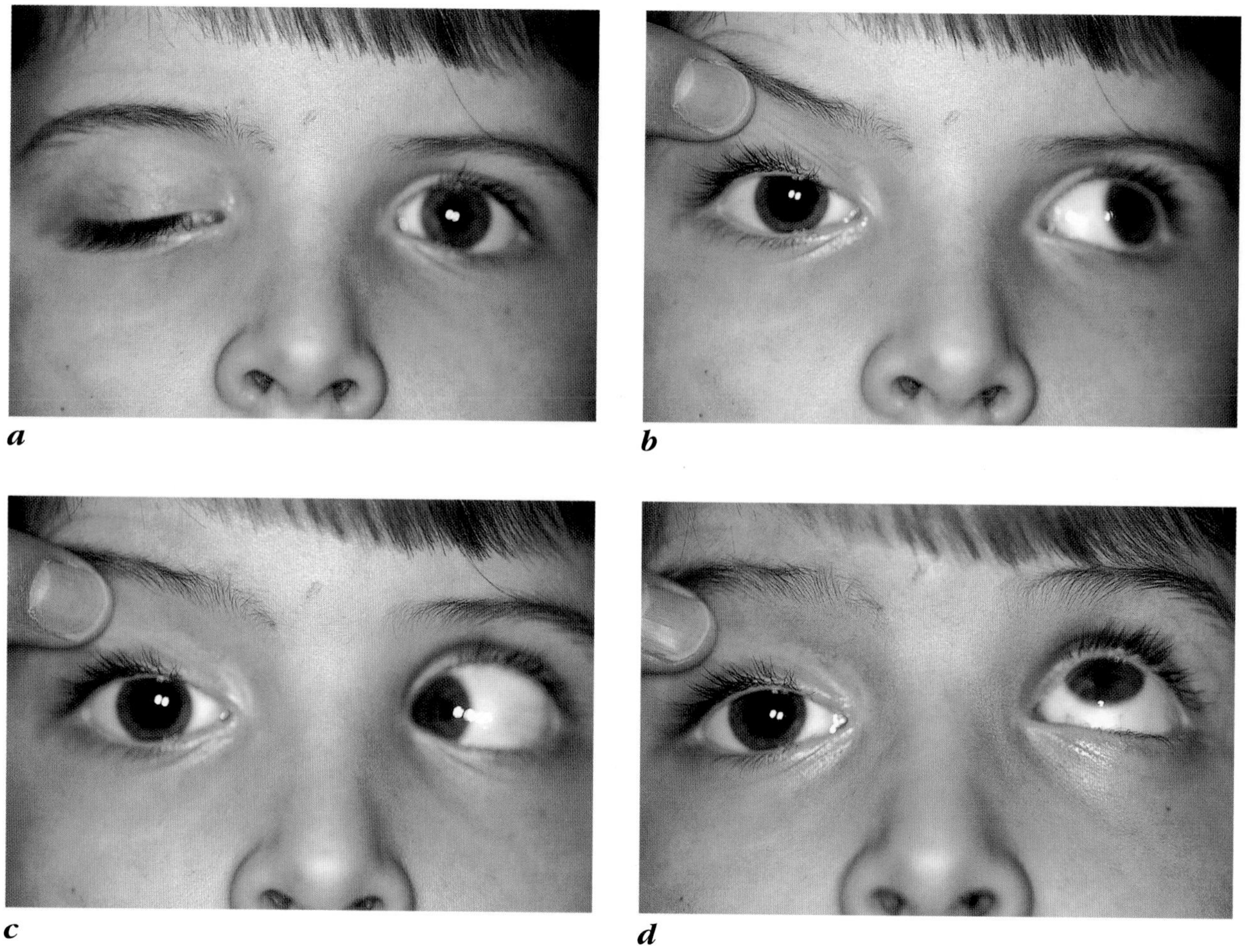

*a*

*b*

*c*

*d*

**Figure 8.9** *Stab wound to the orbit (meat thermometer) causing total ophthalmoplegia but sparing vision.*

possible treatment of 'untreatable' injuries.[1,2] Injuries to the oculomotor nerves (Figs 8.9 and 8.10) usually resolve spontaneously after several months. It is important to remember this when contemplating potential medical or surgical treatment. It is also important to wait the requisite six months before offering surgical correction of these motility defects. In the author's experience, they have all resolved spontaneously after several months.

These large, slowly moving foreign bodies may also cause intracranial injury in addition to total loss of vision (Fig. 8.16). It is important to suspect intracranial penetration in any of these injuries. Vital intracranial structures, specifically the carotid artery and the cavernous sinus, are very close to the orbital apex. Unadvised removal of this foreign body, without first obtaining intracranial exposure to control potential hemorrhage, could be lethal. In treating orbital apical injuries, one should expect and prepare for the worst possible scenario, and be grateful if it does not happen.

## BALLISTICS

The vast majority of orbital injuries caused by rapidly moving foreign bodies result from bullets or pellets.[3,4]

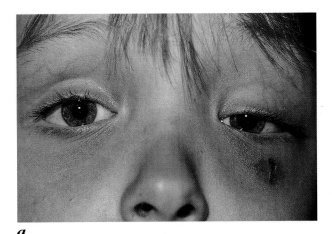

*a*

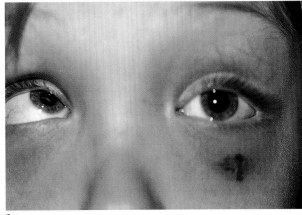

*b*

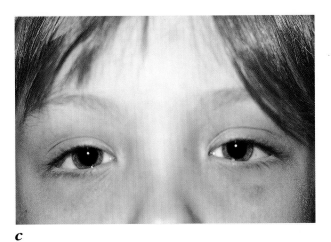

*c*

**Figure 8.10** *Penetrating injury to the inferior orbit causing a partial third-nerve paresis ((a), (b)), totally resolving after 6 weeks (c).*

These injuries are all too common. Again, the destructive effects of a projectile relate to its mass, velocity and fragmentation. Tissue disruption caused by a penetrating object results from a localized crush of tissue in the projectile's path and a momentary stretch of surrounding tissue. The amount of energy generated by a moving object is related to its mass and the square of its velocity. Since velocity is a squared function it is the most important contributor to the energy produced. Velocities of objects penetrating the orbit may be divided into three levels: low, medium and high. The aforementioned knife and stick injuries are examples of low-energy projectiles. The damage inflicted is confined to the direct

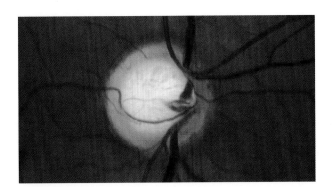

**Figure 8.11** *Normal-appearing optic disc after penetrating injury to the orbital apex and optic nerve.*

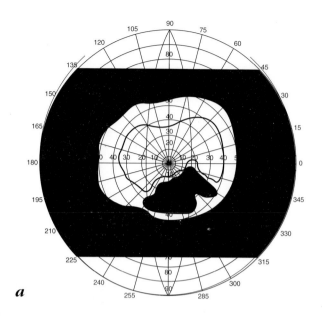

*a*

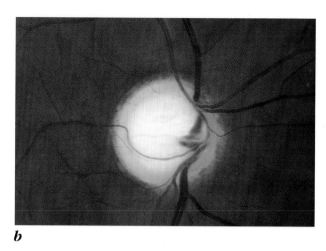

*b*

**Figure 8.12** *Residual visual field defect and optic atrophy. Visual acuity had recovered to 20/100.*

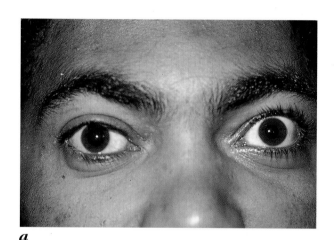

*a*

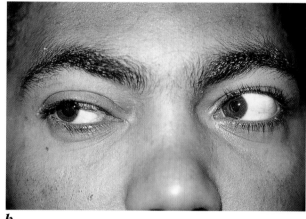

*b*

**Figure 8.13** *Resolution of ptosis and ophthalmoplegia one month after injury.*

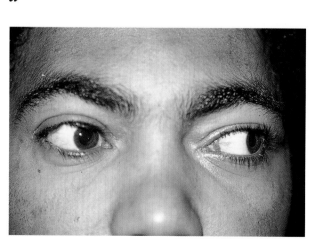

*c*

path of the implement. There is minimal direct damage to adjacent structures. Only objects in the direct path of the projectile are injured initially. Secondary injuries may occur due to edema, infection or ill-advised treatment efforts.

Handguns, airguns and ordinary rifles produce penetrating orbital injuries of medium energy. Ocular damage may be caused by direct penetration (Fig. 8.17). Adjacent structures may also be damaged (Fig. 8.18). Eyes are usually destroyed when struck by these objects, but sometimes they are salvageable. These projectiles have sufficient energy to cause significant ocular or optic nerve damage even when these structures are not in the direct path of the projectile (Fig. 8.19).

High-energy projectiles (military and hunting rifles) cause extensive damage to tissue remote from the path of the projectile. Periorbital injuries caused by these high-energy projectiles are rarely compatible with life and even more rarely evaluated primarily by an ophthalmologist.

Energy can neither be created nor destroyed, only transferred from one form to another, that is, from the projectile to the eye or orbit (Fig. 8.19). This force is equal to the mass of the projectile multiplied by its acceleration or deceleration. The rate of deceleration depends upon the frontal cross-section or sharpness of the projectile. This is determined by the projectile's profile, fragmentation and tumble. The larger the frontal cross-section of the projectile, the more tissue it impacts and the more rapidly it decelerates. More energy is transferred from the projectile to the tissue and more tissue is destroyed. Compare the damage caused by a 12-gauge shotgun blast at short range

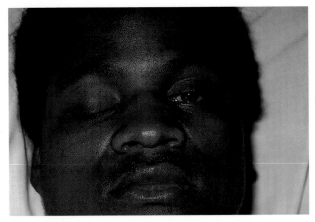

*a*

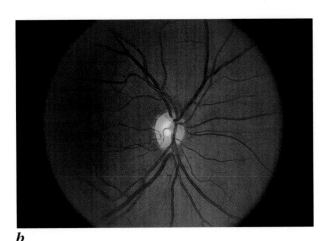

*b*

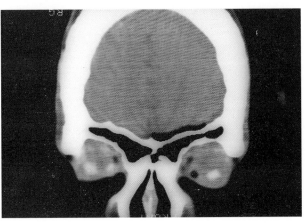

*c*

**Figure 8.14** *Orbital apex syndrome (a) and total amaurosis with a normal-appearing optic disc (b) after a stilleto wound up the nostril with intracranial penetration demonstrated and documented by pneumocephalus on CT scan (c).*

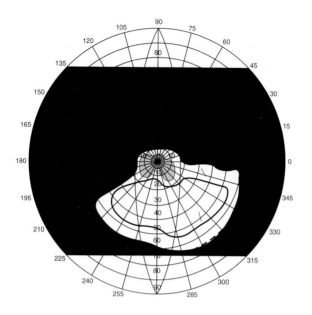

**Figure 8.15** *Visual field after optic canal decompression. Visual acuity improved to 20/50.*

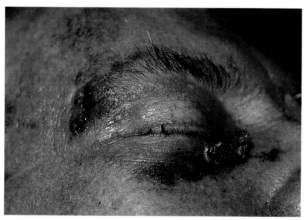

a

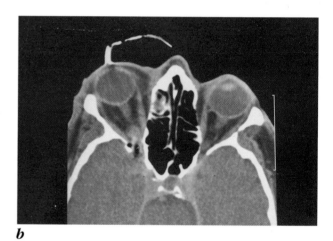

b

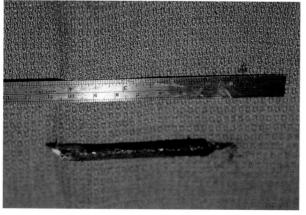

c

**Figure 8.16** *Penetrating injury to orbit (stick) (a) with intracranial involvement evident on CT scan (b). Stick removed after craniotomy and orbitotomy (c).*

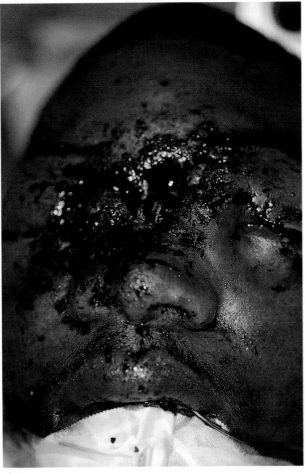

*a*

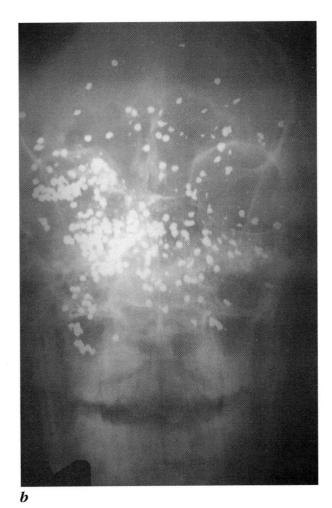

*b*

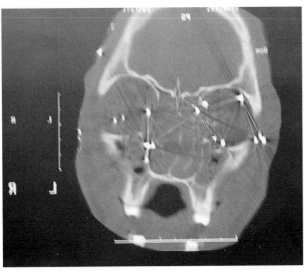

*c*

**Figure 8.17** *Shotgun wound to face destroying both eyes (a). X-ray and CT scan demonstrate extensive pellets in periorbital region (b, c).*

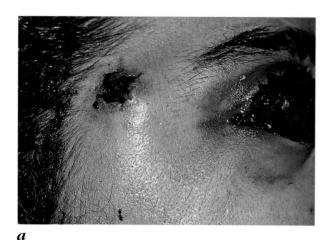
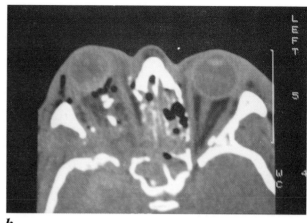

*a*  *b*

**Figure 8.18** *Gunshot wound to orbit (a), sparing the globe but destroying the optic nerve. CT scan demonstrates destruction of optic nerve and orbital structures (b).*

(Fig. 8.17) and a rimfire ·22 bullet (Fig. 8.19). The velocity of the projectiles is the same; but the fragmentation and mass are very different (see Table 8.1).

The most common projectiles causing ocular and orbital injuries are airguns (BBs), bullets, pellets and birdshot. The damage inflicted depends upon the mass, velocity, fragmentation and the path of the projectile. An airgun striking the eye with enough force to rupture the globe causes an irreparable

**Table 8.1** Common projectiles causing orbital injury

| Projectile | Weight (Grams) | Velocity (Feet/second) |
| --- | --- | --- |
| Airgun BB | 5.4 | 150–800 |
| Airgun pellet | 5–9 | 800–900 |
| 'Saturday Night Special' | 38 | 800 |
| 22 Pistol | 30 | 1000 |
| 22 Long | 40 | 1200 |
| 38 caliber | 110 | 800–900 |
| 12-gauge shotgun | 540 | 1200–1400 |

Courtesy of Martin J. Ackler MD, US Army Medical Center, USAMC Director, Wound Ballistics Laboratory, Letterman Army Hospital, San Francisco, California

injury.[5,6] If an airgun is partially deflected by orbital structures, the eye may be salvageable. The child in Fig. 8.20 was struck by an airgun at close range. The airgun was partially deflected by the orbital bone and lodged against the globe underneath the conjunctiva (Fig. 8.20(b)), causing a small hyphema and angle recession glaucoma. If the airgun misses the globe it may lodge in the orbit, causing little damage and visual dysfunction (Figs 8.21 and 8.22). A 12-year-old boy was shot by a friend with a pellet gun (Fig. 8.21). The pellet missed the eye and lodged in the superior orbit (Fig. 8.21 (b)). Visual acuity and extraocular motility was unimpaired. There was no reason to operate upon this patient to remove the pellet. It was causing no damage and would be encapsulated by the orbit and well tolerated. These metallic foreign bodies may be safely left in the orbit unless they are compressing the optic nerve (Fig. 8.22) or otherwise causing visual dysfunction. As a general rule, more damage is caused by trying to locate and remove an intraorbital metallic foreign body than by leaving it alone (Fig. 8.21). The patient in Fig. 8.22 had a similar injury with an airgun. His visual acuity was decreased to bare hand motion, secondary to optic nerve compression at the orbital apex (Fig. 8.22 (b)). High-dose corticosteroids and surgical decompression of the orbital apex and optic canal improved vision to 20/50.

In general, airguns and pellets that penetrate the globe destroy useful vision.[6,7] If they miss the globe,

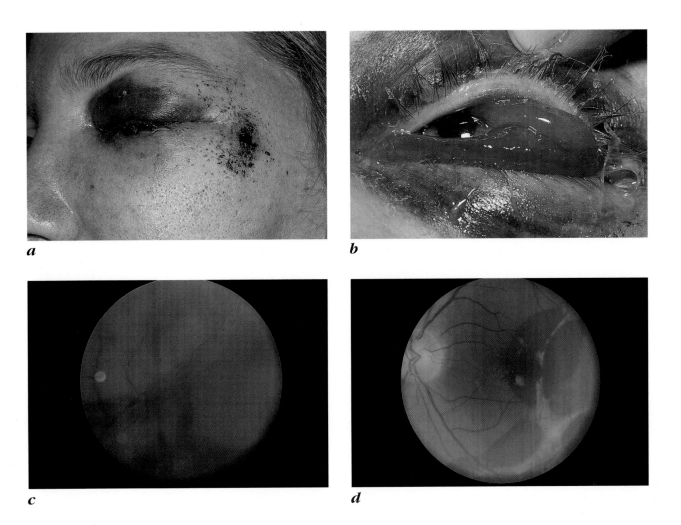

**Figure 8.19** *Self-inflicted gunshot wound (a); bullet missed the globe (b) but extensive chemosis (b) and retinal hemorrhage (c) resulted from the projectile's energy. Red-free photo demonstrates retinal hemorrhage and choroidal tears at the posterior pole (d).*

there is not enough energy dissipated to damage the eye severely, and they usually lodge harmlessly in the orbit (Fig. 8.21). They may also pass through the globe causing an intraocular injury, traverse the orbit and damage the optic nerve, either by direct injury or compression (Fig. 8.23). Rarely, they may cause a compressive optic neuropathy and treatment is necessary. It may be very difficult to find an airgun in the orbital fat and many of these unnecessary surgical expeditions are unsuccessful.

A bullet with a greater mass and velocity may miss the globe but still cause significant damage to the eye due to the greater forces involved (Fig. 8.19). As with pellets and airguns, it is rarely neces-

sary to remove a bullet from the orbit and just as difficult.

Nonmetallic, organic foreign bodies (wood fragments) are more prone to cause an inflammatory reaction or become the nidus of infection. They may also be difficult to localize by computed tomography.[8] Patients with unexplained orbital inflammation should be questioned about the possibility of a remote penetrating orbital injury (Fig. 8.7). Magnetic resonance imaging may be helpful in localizing wooden foreign bodies.[8] Because of their proclivity to act as a nidus of infection, wooden foreign bodies should be removed from the orbit and the wounds copiously irrigated.

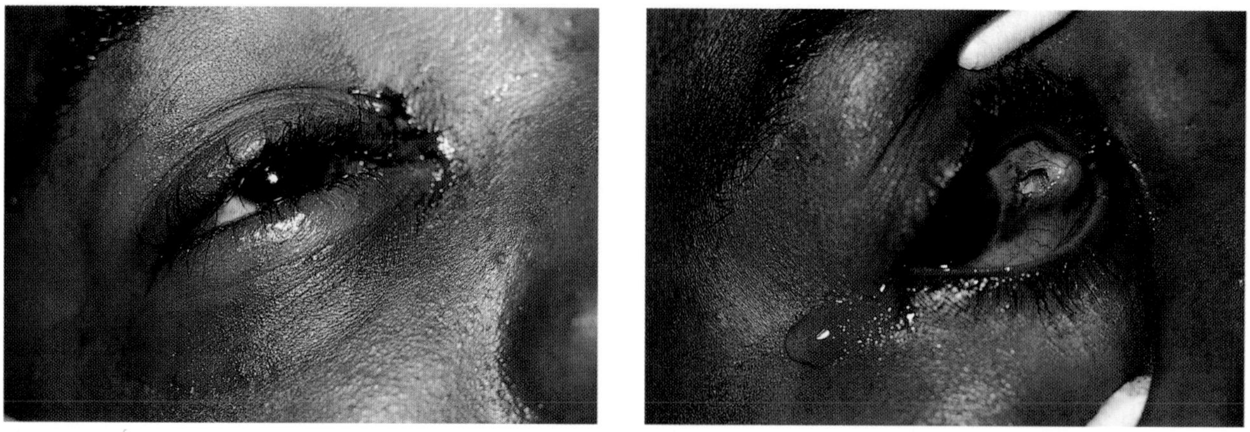

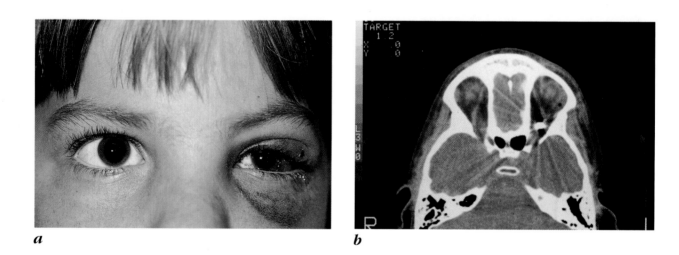

*a*                                        *b*

**Figure 8.20** *Airgun injury to eye. Partial reflection by the medial orbital wall saved the globe from destruction.*

*a*                                        *b*

**Figure 8.21** *A 12-year-old boy shot by a pellet gun (a). The pellet lodged in the superior orbit causing no visual dysfunction (b).*

## EVALUATION OF PENETRATING ORBITAL INJURIES

When confronted with a patient with a projectile injury to the periorbital region, one should expect the worst and appreciate the best result. These injuries should be considered to be intracranial or intraocular until proven otherwise. Computed tomography remains the gold standard for delineating intracranial involvement by periorbital injuries (Fig. 8.16). Intracranial involvement should prompt neurosurgical consultation. The eye should be evaluated. Is the vision normal? If not, why? Is there an afferent pupillary defect indicating optic nerve injury? Is the media clear? Look for evidence for hyphema, subluxation of

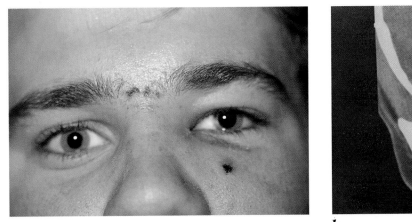
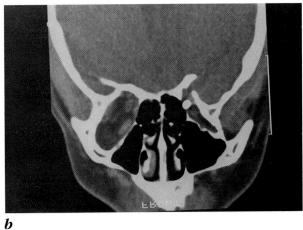

**a**          **b**

**Figure 8.22** *Inferior orbital entry wound (a) caused by an airgun injury. CT scan demonstrating an airgun at the orbital apex causing a compressive optic neuropathy (b).*

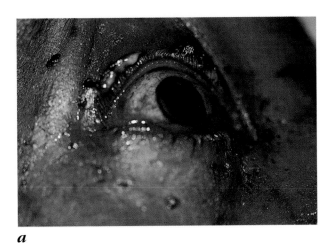
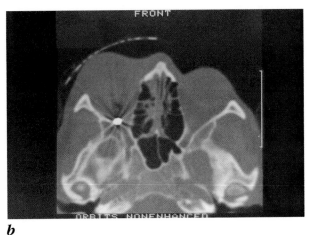

**a**          **b**

**Figure 8.23** *Pellet injury damaging the globe (a) and also injuring the optic nerve at the orbital apex (b).*

the lens, or iris defects that may indicate a penetrating injury. If the media is opacified, review the CT scan. Is there an obvious intraocular foreign body or evidence that the globe has been perforated (Fig. 8.6 (b)) or spared (Fig. 8.4)? Ultrasonography may be very valuable in delineating pathology in an eye with opaque media. If the media is clear, is there evidence for retinal hemorrhage or edema? Is this compatible

with the degree of visual dysfunction? If not, aren't you glad that you detected the afferent pupillary defect prior to dilating the pupils?

If the globe is spared, and there is no intracranial involvement, what should be done with a pellet in the orbit? As discussed previously, no action should be taken unless there is significant compression of the optic nerve, and this is a very uncommon occurrence

(Fig. 8.22). Most pellets lodged in the orbit are best left alone.

Projectile injuries to the eye may involve the anterior segment, posterior segment, or both. These eyes may be completely destroyed or very salvageable. If these eyes are salvageable, they should be patched, shielded and referred to the appropriate subspecialist—often a vitreoretinal surgeon (see Chapter 5). Prophylactic intravenous antibiotics may be given as described in Chapter 1. There is no great urgency in repairing these eyes. Nothing is lost by waiting 12–24 hours until the appropriate surgeon can operate upon the patient in a controlled surgical environment.

# REFERENCES

1 Spoor TC, Hartel WC, Lensink DB. Treatment of traumatic optic neuropathy with corticosteroids. *Am J Ophthalmol* 1990; **110**: 665–9.

2 Spoor TC, Mathog R. Restoration of vision after optic canal decompression following five days of total blindness and megadose corticosteroids. *Arch Ophthalmol* 1986; **104**: 804–6.

3 Frackler ML. Physics of missile injuries. In: McSwain NE, Kerstein MD, eds: *Evaluation and Management of Trauma*, Norwalk, CT: Appleton-Century-Croft, pp 117–25.

4 Chu A, Levine MR. Gunshot wounds of the eye and orbit. *Ophthalmic Surgery* 1989; **20**: 729–36.

5 DeJuan E, Sternberg P, Michels RG. Penetrating ocular injuries. Types of injuries and results. *Ophthalmology* 1983; **90**: 1301–17.

6 Shein P, Engler C, Tielsch JM. The context and consequence of ocular injuries from airguns. *Am J Ophthalmol* 1994; **117**: 501–6.

7 Rudd JC, Jaeger EA, Frietag SK. Traumatically ruptured globes in children. *J Ped Ophthalmol and Strabismus* 1994; **31**: 307–11.

8 Specht CS, Varga JH, Jalali MM et al. Orbitocranial wooden foreign body diagnosed by magnetic resonance imaging. *Surv Ophthalmol* 1992; **36**: 341–4.

# Chapter 9 The inflamed orbit

The key issue in the management of the patient with an inflamed orbit is making an accurate diagnosis and obtaining appropriate neuroimaging studies. These patients are often misdiagnosed when initially examined, with management errors of omission or commission increasing as the clinical course progresses and the patient fails to respond to inappropriate treatment. The following case is illustrative.

A 12-year-old girl (Figs 9.1 (a)–(c)) presented to her optometrist with an inflamed left upper eyelid. The patient was referred to a plastic surgeon and told that she had ptosis and that if it did not resolve in six months he would repair it. The parents sought an

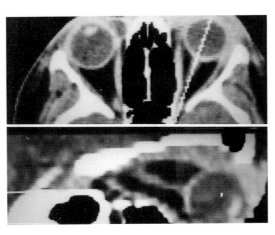

**Figure 9.1 (b)** *CT scan reconstruction demonstrating an enlarged superior rectus-levator complex.*

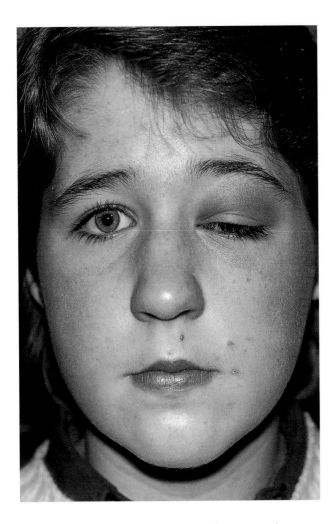

**Figure 9.1 (a)** *Patient presenting with ptosis and an inflamed left upper eyelid and restricted gaze.*

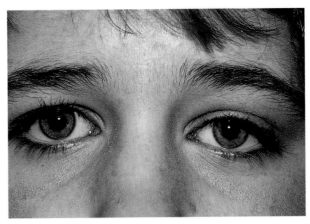

**Figure 9.1 (c)** *Patient in Fig. 9.1 (a) 48 hours after administration of corticosteroids.*

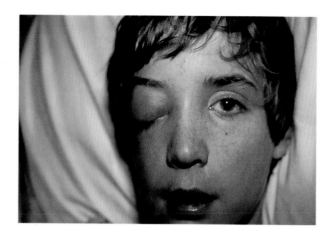

**Figure 9.2** *Patient with an undiagnosed subperiosteal orbital abscess.*

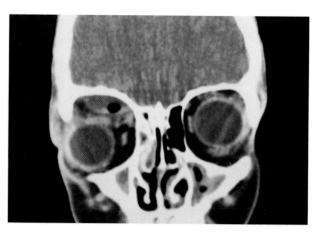

**Figure 9.3** *Coronal CT scan demonstrating the subperiosteal abscess with minimal evidence for ethmoid sinusitis.*

ophthalmologic opinion. The ophthalmologist thought that the child had orbital cellulitis, obtained a CT scan, which was read as negative, and referred the child to an ear, nose and throat (ENT) surgeon for management. The child was hospitalized and treated with a seven-day course of intravenous antibiotics. When she failed to respond a neurologist was consulted who expressed concern that the ptosis might be caused by a manifestation of a cerebral aneurysm, and consulted a neurosurgeon who shared his concern and ordered a four-vessel cerebral angiogram to rule out aneurysm. This too was negative, and the child was discharged from the hospital still with a swollen left upper eyelid. The parents returned to her ophthalmologist who referred her for another opinion. Examination was normal except for an inflamed, ptotic left upper eyelid and restriction of upgaze.

The CT scan was reviewed and thought not to visualize adequately the superior orbit, specifically the superior rectus-levator complex. A repeat CT scan with appropriate reconstructions was obtained and demonstrated an enlargement of the superior rectus-levator complex, confirming the diagnosis of orbital myositis (Fig. 9.1 (b)). Oral corticosteroids were administered, and the patient's condition normalized in 48 hours (Fig. 9.1 (c)).

This case is not unique. The author sees similar cases several times a year. The perpetrators of the misdiagnosis are often otherwise qualified, board-certified ophthalmologists who should know better. The mistakes are often compounded when the physicians involved are not ophthalmologists. This chapter will help the reader to avoid errors of omission and commission when dealing with patients presenting with an acutely inflamed orbit.

The first rule is to decide whether imaging studies are necessary and, if they are, to obtain the appropriate studies, usually a CT scan. Specify the region you wish to examine, that is, the orbit, with thin, 3 mm sections. Obtain the appropriate reconstructions, or better, direct coronal images, and review studies personally. One cannot expect even a superb neuroradiologist to read an orbital study accurately without appropriate clinical information. Is the patient febrile? Are ductions limited? Is the eye pushed up, in, down? Did trauma occur? Is visual function impaired? These scans are difficult enough to interpret without having to do it in a vacuum. The child in Fig. 9.2 was hospitalized on another service for evaluation of an orbital cellulitis presumed secondary to sinusitis. Sinus X-rays and an axial CT scan were compatible with a maxillary and ethmoid sinusitis. Ophthalmologic consultants requested a coronal CT scan better to delineate the orbital structures. The request was denied for fear of inflicting too much radiation upon the child. When the child failed to respond to intravenous antibiotics, an external ethmoidectomy was performed to drain the sinuses. This was minimally productive. The child's

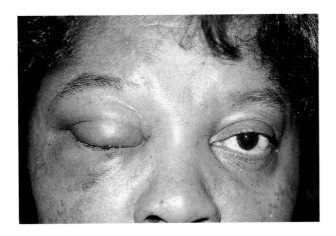

**Figure 9.4** *Preseptal orbital swelling in an afebrile and asymptomatic patient secondary to an adhesive tape allergy.*

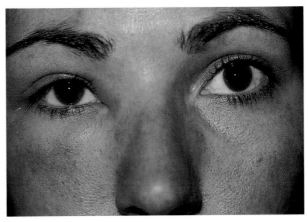

**Figure 9.5** *Preseptal orbital swelling caused by an insect bite to the lower eyelid.*

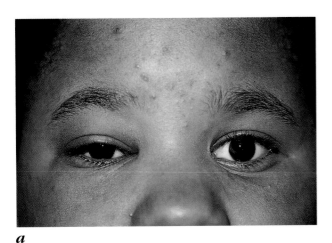

*a*

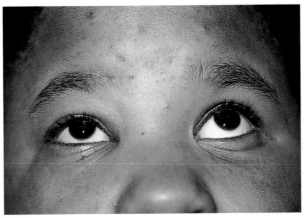

*b*

**Figure 9.6** *Atypical orbital cellulitis. Afebrile patient with a normal WBC presenting with ptosis and upgaze paresis (b).*

condition continued to deteriorate, and the coronal CT scans were reluctantly performed. There was an obvious subperiosteal abscess (Fig. 9.3) which was drained, and the child promptly recovered. It is very difficult to evaluate the orbit properly without adequate imaging studies and appropriate views or reconstructions. These patients may be difficult enough to manage under ideal circumstances: it is important to maximize diagnostic acumen with appropriate studies so that appropriate treatment may be offered.

It is equally important to decide whether the patient needs an imaging study. The lady in Fig. 9.4 was referred for evaluation of a post-traumatic orbital

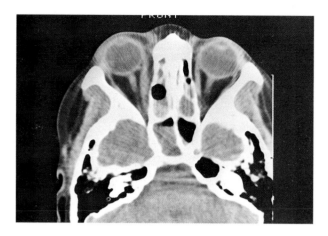

**Figure 9.7** *Axial CT scan demonstrating ethmoiditis and early orbital involvement.*

infection. She was afebrile, only manifesting swelling of the eyelids. She was diagnosed as having an allergic reaction to adhesive tape, and she resolved without treatment, as did the lady in Fig. 9.5 who was referred with early orbital cellulitis and a normal CT scan, vastly overtreating the insect bite on her lower eyelid.

The second rule is to understand one's own limitations of knowledge and experience and to call for help in good time. Patients with orbital disorders may be difficult to diagnose and manage, even by an experienced physician specializing in orbital disease. It is reasonable to seek help from an appropriate consultant.

The most common causes of a proptotic eye and an inflamed orbit are orbital cellulitis, idiopathic orbital inflammation (orbital pseudotumor), dysthyroid orbitopathy, and carotid-cavernous fistulas. Less common causes include retained orbital foreign bodies, dacryoadenitis, and a variety of tumors. Even an experienced clinician has difficulty differentiating these conditions without the benefit of appropriate imaging studies. Differentiating orbital inflammation from orbital cellulitis may be difficult, especially in children. The following cases are illustrative. The patient in Fig. 9.6 presented with ptosis and upgaze paresis in the right eye. Her white bloodcell (WBC) count was normal and she was afebrile. The superior orbit and globe were exquisitely sensitive to palpation. The clinical diagnosis was myositis. A CT scan was obtained (Fig. 9.7) and demonstrated ethmoid sinusitis with early orbital involvement. Treatment with appropriate antibiotics was curative. In contrast, the woman in Fig. 9.8 was febrile and had an elevated WBC count. The left eye was proptotic and ductions were limited (Fig. 9.8 (b)). The clinical diagnosis was orbital cellulitis. A CT scan (Fig. 9.9)

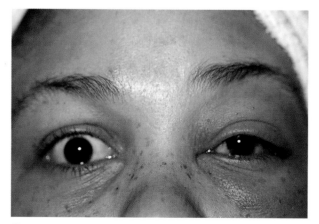

*a*

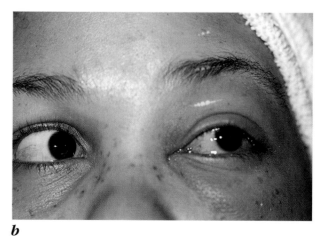

*b*

**Figure 9.8** *Atypical orbital myositis. Febrile patient with elevated WBC presenting with pain, ptosis and decreased ocular abduction (b).*

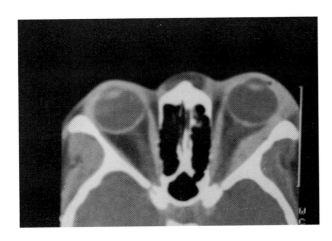

**Figure 9.9** *CT scan demonstrating enlargement of the lateral rectus muscle and normal sinuses.*

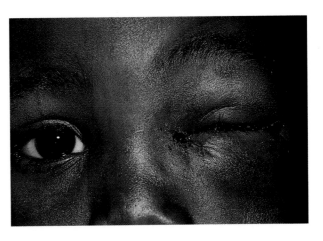

**Figure 9.10** *Dacryocystitis with preseptal orbital involvement. Lacrimal sac involvement is diagnostic.*

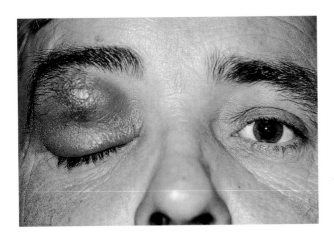

**Figure 9.11** *Preseptal cellulitis.*

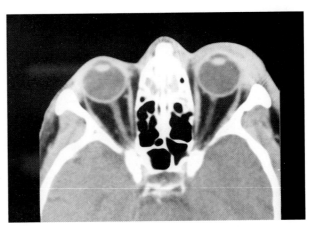

**Figure 9.12** *CT scan of preseptal cellulitis demonstrates entire inflammatory process confined anterior of the orbital septum.*

was obtained and demonstrated enlargement of the lateral rectus muscle and normal sinuses. The diagnosis was the myositic variant of idiopathic orbital inflammation, and treatment with corticosteroids was curative. These cases demonstrate that appropriate computerized tomography is essential to differentiate orbital cellulitis from orbital inflammation, even by experienced clinicians.

## ORBITAL INFECTIONS

Orbital infections may result from trauma, with or without retained orbital foreign bodies, facial or dental infections, adjacent sinusitis or dacryocystitis (Fig. 9.10). These infections are usually preseptal and may be distinguished from orbital cellulitis (postseptal)

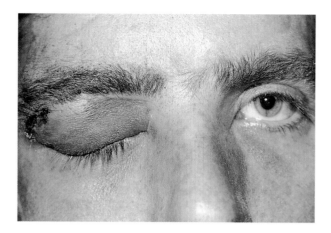

**Figure 9.13** *Preseptal orbital cellulitis due to a foreign body.*

eyelid is usually initially involved, with progression to the upper and lower eyelids. The eye is usually uninvolved, but conjunctival chemosis may occur with progression. Since the infection is periorbital or anterior to the orbital septum (Fig. 9.12), visual function—acuity, pupils and extraocular motility—is not affected. This inflammatory edema results from congestion of venous return and needs to be differentiated from edema secondary to an allergic reaction (Figs 9.4 and 9.5) and eyelid and anterior orbital infections due to foreign bodies, trauma (Fig. 9.13) and drainage of an adjacent sinus infection into the anterior orbit (Fig. 9.14). This differentiation is important because preseptal cellulitis due to ethmoid sinusitis can progress to a more severe orbital infection, whereas preseptal cellulitis due to trauma, foreign body or contiguous spread from a nonsinus source usually remains confined to the preseptal space. These infections may look terrible, but usually respond to antibiotics and debridement and spare the deep orbit (Figs 9.15 and 9.16).

Chandler et al.[1] classified orbital cellulitis secondary to sinusitis as a continuum of severity. Preseptal cellulitis leads to orbital cellulitis which progresses to a subperiosteal abscess to an intraorbital abscess to cavernous sinus thrombosis. As mentioned above, preseptal cellulitis represents inflammatory edema of the eyelids and periorbital region (Fig. 9.11). In true orbital cellulitis, the orbit itself is infiltrated posterior to the orbital septum. This represents an expanding mass in a closed space with

by the lack of systemic signs, normal visual acuity and motility function. If the latter are abnormal, the infection is by definition postseptal orbital cellulitis. Orbital infections are often due to adjacent sinusitis and may also be preseptal or postseptal. Preseptal cellulitis (Fig. 9.11) is inflammatory edema characterized by swelling of the eyelids and orbit anterior to the orbital septum. The medial portion of the upper

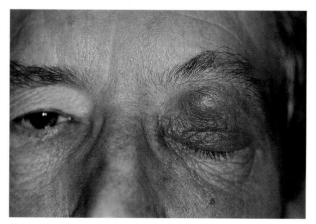

*a*

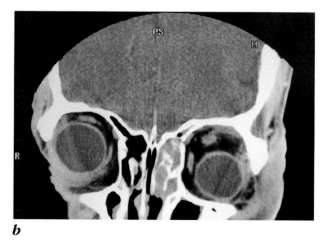

*b*

**Figure 9.14** *Eyelid abscess secondary to fronto-ethmoid sinusitis draining into eyelid (b).*

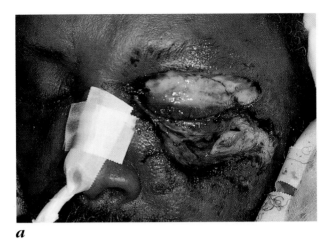

*a*

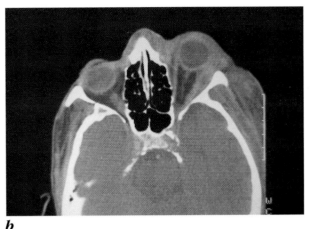

*b*

Figure 9.15 *Severe preseptal infection after eyelid trauma. CT scan demonstrates sparing of the postseptal deep orbit (b). Eventual recovery after antibiotics and debridement (c).*

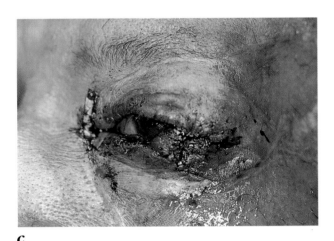

*c*

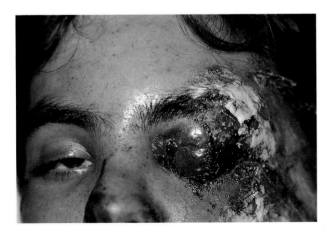

Figure 9.16 *Severe post-traumatic preseptal infection sparing the deep orbit.*

resultant proptosis, extraocular motility and visual dysfunction (Figs 9.17 (a)–(c)).

An abscess within the subperiosteal space may displace the globe and compress apical orbital structures causing proptosis and visual loss (Fig. 9.18). Progression of orbital cellulitis or spread of a subperiosteal abscess may lead to an intraorbital abscess (Fig. 9.19). These patients present with proptosis, motility and visual dysfunction, and systemic toxicity. Cavernous sinus thrombosis is the ultimate extension of orbital cellulitis. These patients are profoundly ill with severe visual dysfunction. The eye may be blind, the globe frozen secondary to involvement of the oculomotor nerves in the cavernous sinus (Fig. 9.20). Sinus and orbital infections may also cause adjacent cerebral abscesses or subdural empyema. These patients have a very significant morbidity, and

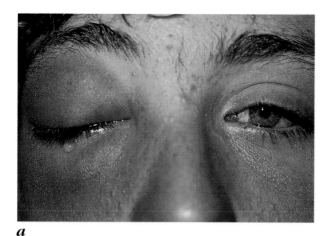

*a*

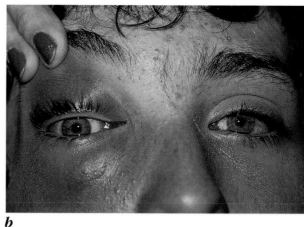

*b*

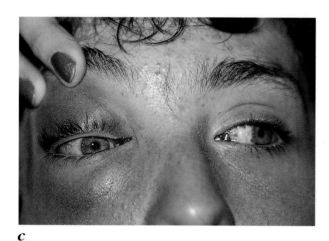

*c*

**Figure 9.17** *Orbital cellulitis: preseptal inflammation now accompanied by proptosis, restricted adduction and subtle pupillary dilatation.*

prompt diagnosis may be life-saving. It is important to remember that in the preantibiotic era, 25% of patients with orbital cellulitis died and another 25% were blinded by their infection. Orbital infections are potentially lethal and blinding.

## TREATMENT

Treatment of orbital cellulitis is influenced by the patient's age, visual function, presumed etiology of the infection, and presence or absence of an abscess on imaging studies. A CT scan should be promptly obtained on any patient with a presumed orbital infection. Axial and coronal studies should be done to localize the abscess properly. Preseptal cellulitis should be treated with intravenous antibiotics, especially if it is caused by an adjacent sinusitis, for it may progress to postseptal involvement. Postseptal or true orbital cellulitis should be treated aggressively with meningeal doses of intravenous antibiotics. Abscesses need to be promptly drained if there is evidence for optic nerve dysfunction (decreased vision and an afferent pupillary defect). Although there are some recent data documenting that some subperiosteal abscesses may respond to intravenous antibiotics,[2,3] in the face of visual dysfunction most surgeons would elect drainage.

Children need to be treated differently from adults, taking into consideration the susceptibility of children under 5 years of age to infection by *Haemophilus influenzae*.[4] The author's group consider all children under 12 years of age as if they were susceptible to *H. influenzae* and choose antibiotics accordingly. A

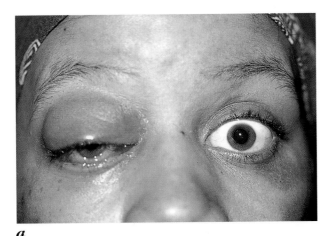

*a*

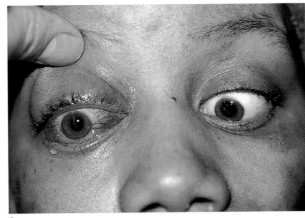

*b*

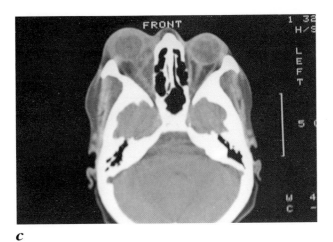

*c*

**Figure 9.18** *More advanced orbital cellulitis demonstrates proptosis, obvious pupillary dilatation and ophthalmoplegia. CT scan demonstrates a subperiosteal abscess (c).*

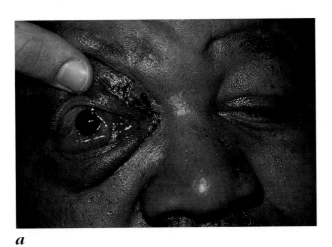

*a*

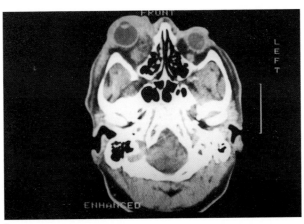

*b*

**Figure 9.19** *Orbital cellulitis: proptosis, chemosis, ophthalmoplegia and visual loss. CT scan demonstrates an intraorbital abscess (b).*

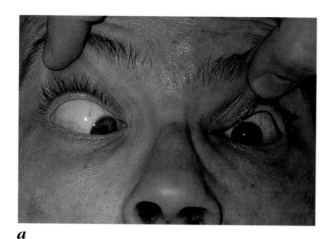

*a*

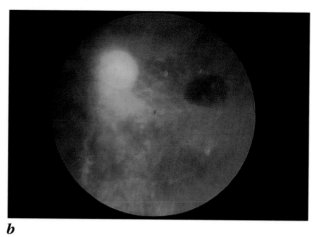

*b*

**Figure 9.20** *Cavernous sinus thrombosis with total ophthalmoplegia and blindness due to an ophthalmic artery infarction (b).*

second-generation cephalosporin, cefuroxamine, is effective against most gram-positive cocci, oral anaerobes and *H. influenzae*. Recommended dosage is 100 mg/kg daily in three or four divided doses. Cefuroxamine also penetrates soft tissue, bone and cerebrospinal fluid (CSF) well and is an excellent drug for these patients.

In adults, high-dose antibiotic therapy should be administered with coverage for penicillin-resistant cocci, anaerobes and gram-negatives. Gram-negative infections are of special concern in patients with diabetes mellitus. A classic regimen includes methicilline 2 g every 6 hours and gentamycin 80 mg every 8 hours with the dose adjusted as per the pharmacokinetic determinations of peak and trough levels. A more modern regimen would consist of intravenous ciprofloxacin—1 g every 12 hours—and ceftazidime—1 g every 12 hours.

The issue of overutilization of new antibiotics and selection of resistant organisms is best discussed elsewhere. Antibiotic regimens will vary with location, suspected organisms and mechanism of injury. Table 9.1 depicts some typical treatment regimens for both adults and children for quick reference.

**Table 9.1**  Antibiotic treatment of orbital cellulitis

*Children*
Cefuroxime 100 mg/kg daily in three divided doses

*Adults*
Ciprofloxacin 1 gm q12h
Ceftazidime 1 gm q12h
*or*
Methacillin 2 g q6h
Gentamycin 80 mg q8h

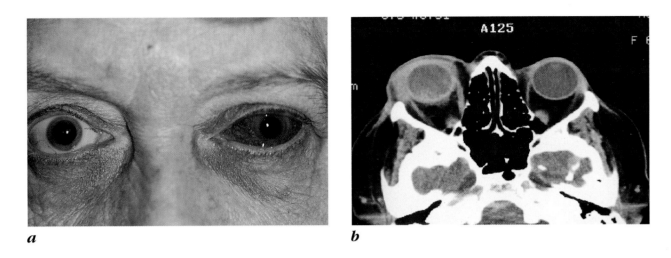

**Figure 9.21** *Acute periscleritis with CT evidence for diffuse periscleral inflammation (b).*

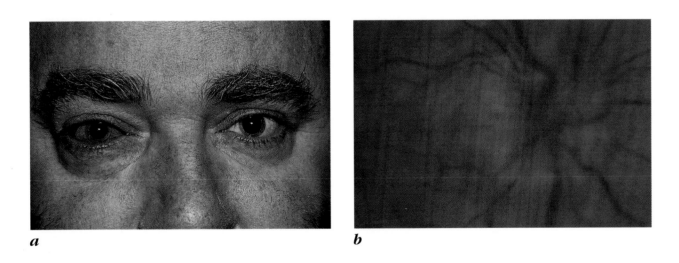

**Figure 9.22** *Periscleritis combined with swelling of the optic disc secondary to perineural inflammation.*

## IDIOPATHIC ORBITAL INFLAMMATION

In the early days of CT scanning orbital pseudotumor was renamed idiopathic orbital inflammation, and Trokel et al.[5] used CT findings to subdivide it into four distinct entities. These are periscleritis: diffuse enhancement of the globe (Fig. 9.21); perineuritis: enhancement of the optic nerve sparing vision (Fig. 9.22); dacryoadenitis: enlargement and enhancement of the lacrimal gland (Fig. 9.23); myositis: enlargement and enhancement of one or more extraocular muscles (Fig. 9.24). Patients with acute dysthyroid orbitopathy may mimic orbital myositis, are often less

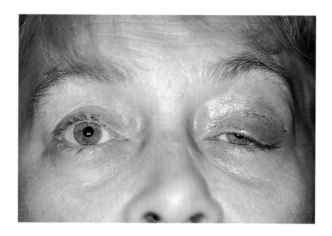

**Figure 9.23** *Dacryoadenitis demonstrating a distinctive S-shaped ptosis secondary to lacrimal gland enlargement.*

Orbital inflammation may also be classified as anterior and posterior. Patients with anterior inflammation will present with a red, painful eye (Figs 9.21, 9.22, 9.24). Patients with posterior inflammation may have pain and motility or visual dysfunction, but may not have obvious peribulbar inflammation (Fig. 9.26). As with patients with other forms of orbital inflammation, CT scanning is essential to make the diagnosis prior to commencing treatment with systemic corticosteroids.

The author utilizes prednisone or its methylprednisolone equivalent 80 mg daily for two weeks. Response is usually dramatic, with relief of pain and normalization of function occurring in 24–48 hours. Steroids are then tapered in 20 mg decrements every two weeks. When symptoms and signs recur with steroid taper, an unusual form of orbital inflammation like Wegener's granulomatosis, occult fungal infection, or neoplasm should be considered.

tender, have telltale eyelid retraction and a distinctive clinical and CT appearance (Fig. 9.25). Patients may also present with any combination of these findings. The common denominator is that these patients have a painful, red eye that must be differentiated from an acute orbital infection.

## CAROTID-CAVERNOUS FISTULA

A carotid-cavernous fistula is an abnormal communication between the intracavernous carotid artery and the cavernous sinus. Trauma usually results in direct shunts between the carotid artery and the cavernous

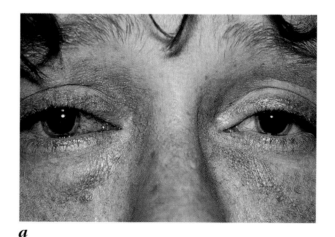

*a*

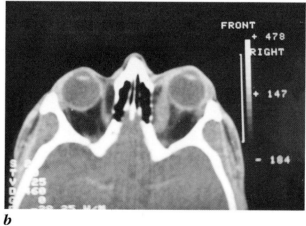

*b*

**Figure 9.24** *Orbital myositis manifesting an inflamed eye, an adduction deficit and an enlarged medial rectus on CT (b).*

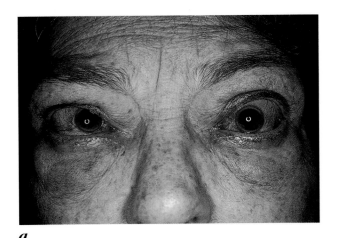

*a*

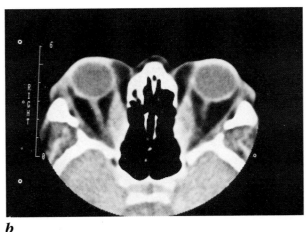

*b*

**Figure 9.25** *Acute orbital inflammation due to dysthyroid orbitopathy. Note the telltale eyelid retraction and distinctive appearance of the enlarged muscle's tendons on CT scan (b).*

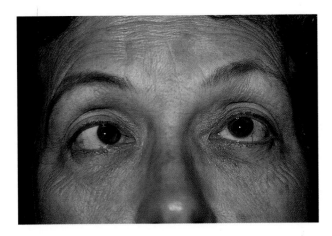

**Figure 9.26** *Patient with a painful left sixth-nerve palsy secondary to posterior orbital inflammation.*

sinus. These represent high-flow fistulas; their presentation is rarely subtle. Patients present with early signs and symptoms including pulsatile proptosis, ocular and orbital erythema, chemosis, arteriolization of the conjunctival vessels, diplopia, headaches, noises in the head, and visual loss (Figs

9.27 and 9.28). More subtle dural-based fistulas tend to occur spontaneously and need be included in the differential diagnosis of the chronically red eye (Fig. 9.29).

The key to diagnosing carotid-cavernous fistulas is thinking of the diagnosis. The patient presenting in the setting of trauma may have an obvious carotid-cavernous fistula on presentation (Fig. 9.28) or may be normal for several days after trauma and then spontaneously develop a carotid-cavernous fistula (Fig. 9.27). Computerized tomography demonstrates enlargement of the superior ophthalmic vein, cavernous sinus (Fig. 9.29 (b)). The extraocular muscles may be enlarged, and the orbital contents appear edematous (Fig. 9.27 (b) and 9.28 (b)).

These patients are best managed in concert with a neurosurgeon and interventional neuroradiologist. Ninety percent of traumatic carotid-cavernous fistulas may be cured by intra-arterial placement of a detachable balloon to occlude the fistula. The remaining patients may require a transvenous approach through the superior ophthalmic vein.[6]

Traumatic optic neuropathy may accompany a carotid-cavernous fistula, especially in patients with extensive mid-face or base-of-brain fractures. The engorged cavernous sinus may herniate into the sphenoid sinus. Inadvertent entry during extracranial optic canal decompression may result in a very extensive bleeding diathesis.

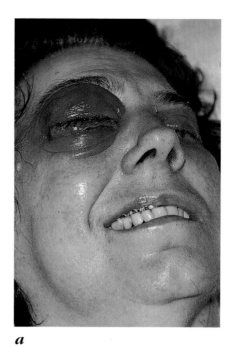

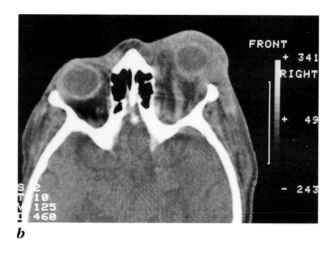

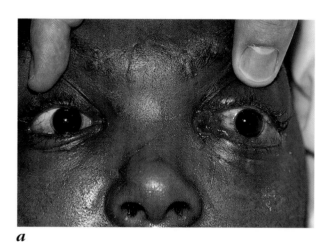

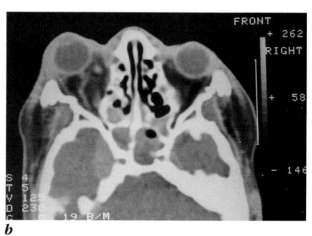

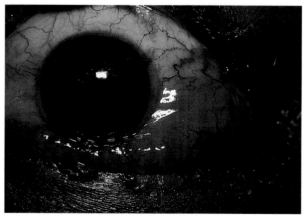

**Figure 9.27** *Obvious carotid-cavernous fistula appearing several days after cranial trauma. CT scan demonstrates marked swelling of the eye and eyelids, proptosis and elongation and enlargement of the superior ophthalmic vein (b).*

**Figure 9.28** *Carotid-cavernous fistula after cranial and facial trauma, with arterialization of the conjunctival vessels (b). CT scan demonstrates periocular edema, enlargement of the superior ophthalmic vein and cavernous sinus (c).*

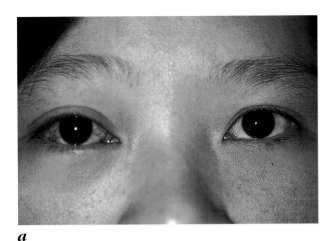

*a*

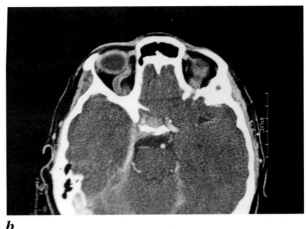

*b*

**Figure 9.29** *Dural cavernous fistula managed as chronic conjunctivitis. An enlarged superior ophthalmic vein on CT scan alerted the clinician to the proper diagnosis (b).*

## ORBITAL HEMORRHAGES

As with orbital infections, hemorrhages may be either preseptal, postseptal and confined behind the orbital septum, or subperiosteal. Preseptal orbital hemorrhages are confined to the eyelids and brow. They may look terrible (Fig. 9.30) but they are benign. They may be accompanied by a concomitant orbital floor or medial wall fracture (Fig. 9.31). Vision is usually unimpaired and the hemorrhage usually resolves spontaneously. A loculated area of hemorrhage may be drained surgically or aspirated with a 22-gauge needle to speed resolution. It is important to document visual acuity and pupillary reactions: for example, is there an afferent pupillary defect? In patients with preseptal orbital hemorrhage, the blunt injury that caused the hemorrhage may have also caused injury to the optic nerve and a concomitant optic neuropathy (Fig. 9.32) (see Chapter 11). Documentation of visual function is important. Although there is no firm consensus as to the appropriate medical or surgical management of optic nerve injuries, the potential legal implications of not assessing visual function are obvious.

## SUBPERIOSTEAL HEMORRHAGES

Subperiosteal hemorrhages are caused by avulsion of the penetrating vessels entering the periorbita (dura)

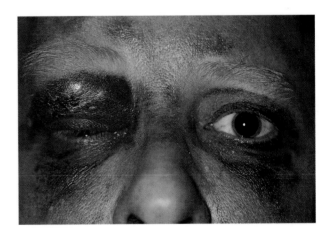

**Figure 9.30** *Preseptal orbital hemorrhage with normal ocular function.*

from the adjacent bone. This is similar to an epidermal hematoma. As the hemorrhage progresses it acts as an expanding mass, causing proptosis, displacement of the globe, extraocular motility dysfunction, and visual loss (Fig. 9.33). Computerized tomography with coronal views is diagnostic, demonstrating an extraconal blood density mass in the subperiosteal

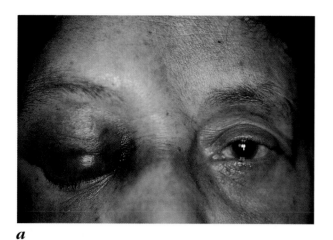

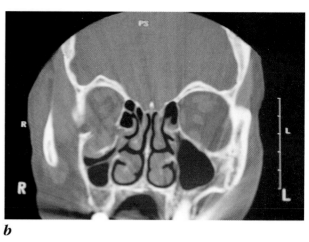

*a*        *b*

**Figure 9.31** *Preseptal orbital hemorrhage accompanied by a large orbital floor fracture (b) whose presence may be obscured by the hemorrhage and edema.*

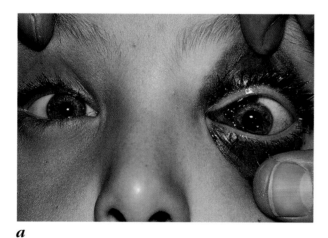

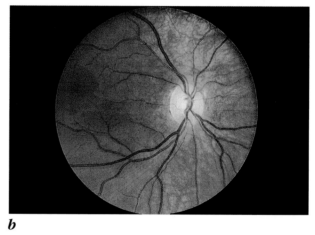

*a*        *b*

**Figure 9.32** *An 11-year-old boy struck in the eye with a pool cue with resultant mydriasis, abduction deficit and a traumatic optic neuropathy. Optic atrophy (b) and a superior altitudinal visual field occurred in spite of diagnosis and treatment with megadose corticosteroids.*

space (Fig. 9.33 (b)). Small hemorrhages causing no visual dysfunction may reabsorb spontaneously; larger hemorrhages causing visual dysfunction and disfigurement should be drained.

Drainage may be easily accomplished by making an incision through the skin, orbicularis and periosteum, dissecting the periosteum from the orbital rim with a Freer elevator (Stortz Instruments, St Louis, MO) and entering the subperiosteal space. The hemorrhage may be evacuated with suction and bleeding controlled with bone wax or bipolar cautery, depending upon whether it is arising from the emissary vessels from the bone or the periorbita. Symptoms rapidly resolve after evacuation of the hemorrhage (Fig. 9.33 (c)).

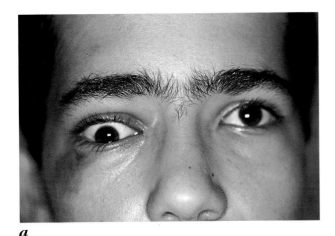

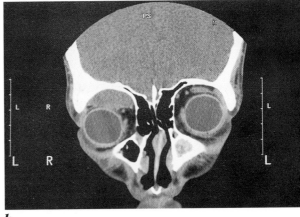

*a*

*b*

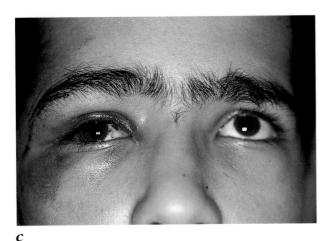

*c*

**Figure 9.33** *A 15-year-old boy struck in the right orbit referred with a presumed orbital fracture. CT scan (b) demonstrates a large, superior, subperiosteal orbital hemorrhage. Appearance one week after surgical evacuation (c).*

# POSTSEPTAL ORBITAL HEMORRHAGES

Treatment of diffuse orbital hemorrhages may be expectant or emergent. Hemorrhages causing mild proptosis, motility dysfunction, and mildly elevated intraocular pressure may be managed by observation. They often resolve spontaneously with no permanent sequelae (Fig. 9.34). They may be relatively asymptomatic causing subtle proptosis and minimal visual dysfunction. No treatment is necessary, and spontaneous resolution is the rule (Fig. 9.34).

Orbital hemorrhages causing decreased visual function, either by compressing the optic nerve or compromising retinal circulation, should be treated expeditiously. An emergent canthotomy and cantholysis should be performed under local anesthetic.

This often results in adequate decompression to restore or maintain retinal perfusion. The most common mistake seen is performance of an inadequate canthotomy/cantholysis. These must be performed aggressively. At the conclusion, the eyelids should be freely disinserted from the lateral orbital rim.

A technique has been described to decompress the orbital floor with a hemostat passed through the inferior fornix and fracturing the orbital floor.[7] This is usually not necessary if an adequate canthotomy/ cantholysis has been performed. It may also be nearly impossible in individuals with thick orbital floors. These thick floors may be very evident on CT scan; however, if these patients are being managed expeditiously, the canthotomy/cantholysis will be performed prior to obtaining the CT scan.

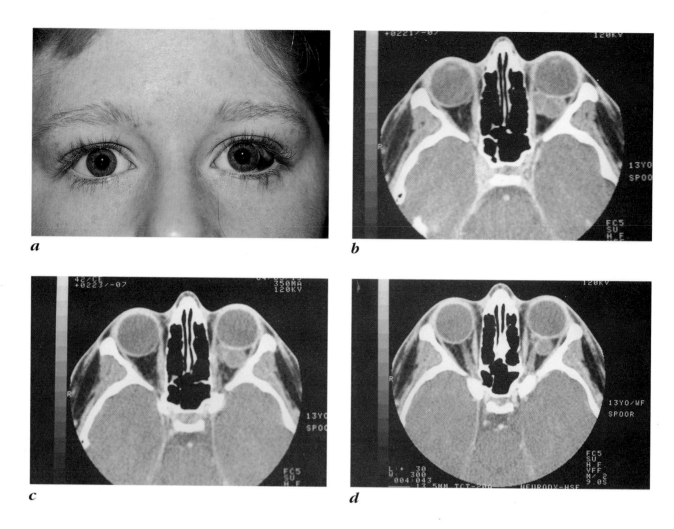

*a*

*b*

*c*

*d*

**Figure 9.34** *Asymptomatic, circumscribed orbital hemorrhage presenting as proptosis and a subconjunctival hemorrhage. CT scan demonstrates an intraconal mass (b) resolving over several months (c, d).*

Decompression of the orbital floor with a hemostat or at surgery may be accomplished if necessary.

Orbital hemorrhages may also be well circumscribed and drainage may be carried out with a 22-gauge needle. Computed tomography or orbital ultrasonography should be carried out to localize the hemorrhage prior to sticking a needle blindly into the orbit. Aspiration of the blood-filled cyst may temporize or resolve the problem (Fig. 9.35).

Rarely, a hemorrhage may be confined to the vaginal space surrounding the intraorbital optic nerve. A small amount of bleeding confined to a very small potential space may cause devastating visual loss. These patients present with visual loss and an afferent pupillary defect out of proportion to the degree of hemorrhage evident (Fig. 9.36 (a)). Fundus examination may demonstrate an apparent venous stasis retinopathy (Fig. 9.36 (b)). CT scan is diagnostic, demonstrating an enlarged optic nerve with blood density (Fig. 9.36 (c)). Emergent optic nerve sheath

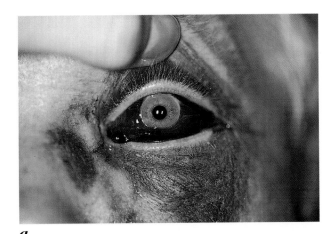

*a*

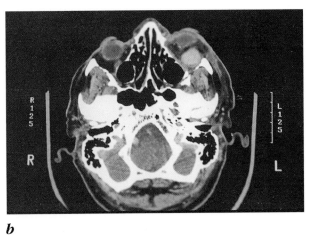

*b*

**Figure 9.35** *Traumatic, well circumscribed orbital hemorrhage (a) causing visual loss, localized by CT scan (b) and aspirated with a 22-gauge needle (c).*

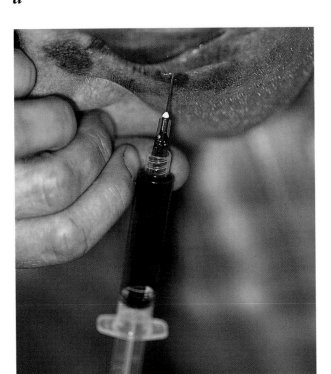

*c*

decompression drains the blood, relieves the pressure upon the optic nerve fibers, and may be sight-saving.

## OTHER CAUSES OF ORBITAL HEMORRHAGES

Spontaneous orbital hemorrhages may occur in the absence of obvious trauma; however, a history of minor trauma can often be elicited (Fig. 9.34). If the patient with an orbital hemorrhage steadfastly denies any history of even trivial trauma, suspect leukemia (Fig. 9.37) or lymphoma. Metastatic prosthetic carcinoma may present as an inflamed, hemorrhagic orbit (Fig. 9.38). If a child presents with an orbital hemorrhage, without a plausible etiology, suspect child abuse until proven otherwise, although lymphangiomas may often present with a spontaneous orbital hemorrhage and proptosis (Fig. 9.39).

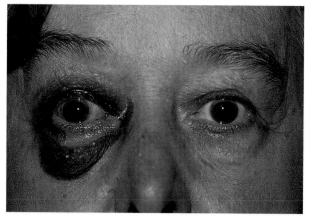

*a*

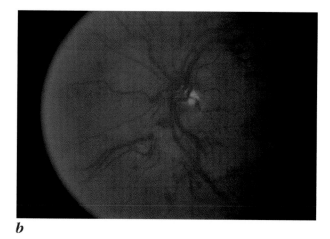

*b*

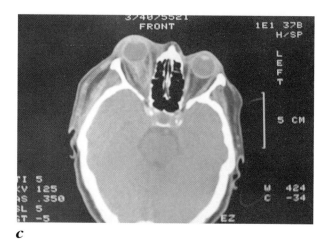

*c*

**Figure 9.36** *Patient struck in the eye with a fist presenting with a blind eye. Fundus photo demonstrating venous stasis retinopathy out of proportion to the degree of visual loss and the amaurotic pupil (b). CT scan demonstrating an optic nerve sheath hemorrhage compressing the optic nerve (c).*

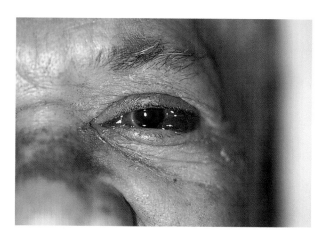

**Figure 9.37** *Patient presenting with spontaneous hyphema, and subconjunctival and orbital hemorrhage secondary to pancytopenia caused by leukemia.*

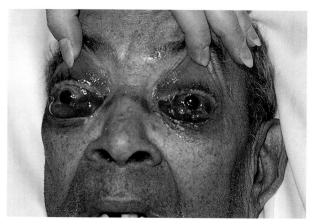

**Figure 9.38** *Bilateral orbital and subconjunctival hemorrhages in patient with known metastatic prostate carcinoma.*

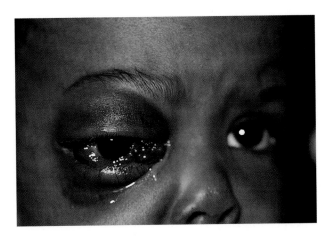

**Figure 9.39** *Spontaneous orbital hemorrhage in a child may represent a lymphangioma/varix; however, child abuse should be suspected if there is no CT evidence for tumour.*

# REFERENCES

1   Chandler JR, Langenbranner, DJ, Stevens ER. The pathogenesis of orbital complications in acute sinusitis. *Laryngoscope* 1970; **80**: 1414–21.

2   Harris GJ. Age as a factor in the bacteriology and response to treatment of subperiosteal abscess of the orbit. *Trans Am Ophthalmol Soc* 1993; **91**: 441–516.

3   Harris GJ. Subperiosteal abscess of the orbit. Age as a factor in the bacteriology and response to treatment. *Ophthalmology* 1994; **101**: 585–95.

4   Williams SR, Carruth JA. Orbital infection secondary to sinusitis in children: diagnosis and management. *Clin Otolaryngol (Eng.)* 1992; **17**: 550–7.

5   Trokel SL, Hilal SK. Recognition and differential diagnosis of enlarged extraocular muscles in computed tomography. *Am J Ophthalmol* 1979; **87**: 503.

6   Jiminez DE, Gibbs SR. Carotid-cavernous sinus fistula in craniofacial trauma. *J Cranio-maxillofacial Trauma* 1995; **1**: 7–15.

7   Liu D. A simplified technique of orbital decompression for severe retrobulbar hemorrhage. *Am J Ophthalmol* 1993; **116**: 34–7.

# *Chapter 10* **Orbital fractures**

*Thomas C Spoor and John McHenry*

Typical orbital fractures evaluated and treated by an ophthalmologist include pure blowout fractures of the orbital floor, medial orbital wall fractures and trimalar fractures. Patients often have a combination of fractures depending on the type and severity of their injuries.

Orbital floor fractures may be isolated or occur in combination with medial orbital wall fractures. The classic injury is a fist or a ball striking the anterior orbit, compressing the eye into the orbit (Fig. 10.1).[1] The thin orbital floor fractures medial to the infraorbital neurovascular bundle. The even thinner medial orbital wall may or may not be involved. Orbital floor fractures may be asymptomatic, but usually are accompanied by some combination of paresthesias over the distribution of the infraorbital nerve, enophthalmos, or diplopia with or without entrapment of the inferior rectus muscle or its septae. Fractures of the medial orbital wall are often accompanied by orbital emphysema (Fig. 10.2 (a) and (b)).

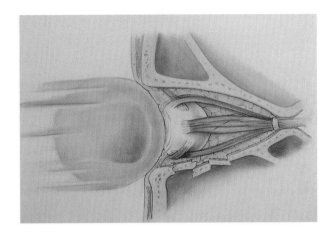

**Figure 10.1** *The globe is struck by an object larger than the orbital opening, in this case a tennis ball. The eye is compressed into the orbit and the resultant energy fractures the thin medial wall and orbital floor.*

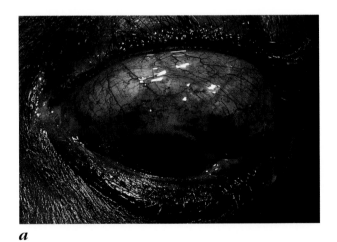

*a*

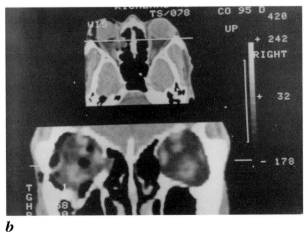

*b*

**Figure 10.2** *Severe orbital emphysema (a) secondary to a medial orbital wall fracture. CT scan (b) demonstrating medial orbital wall fracture and intraorbital air.*

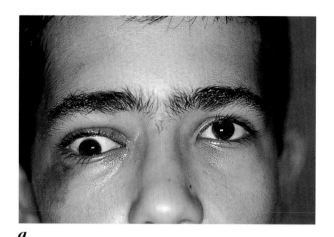
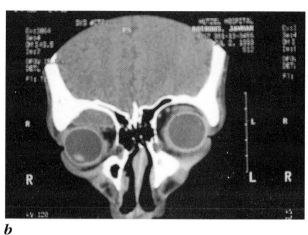

*a*                         *b*

**Figure 10.3** *Globe ptosis and proptosis after blunt trauma (a). CT scan demonstrating a superior subperiosteal hemorrhage (b).*

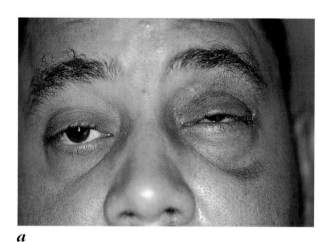
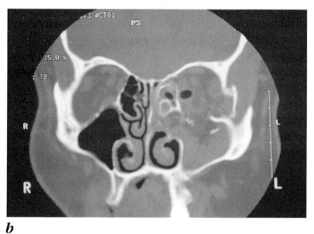

*a*                         *b*

**Figure 10.4** *Patients with large orbital floor fractures may be initially enophthalmic, or enophthalmos may be masked by orbital swelling and hemorrhages (a). CT scan demonstrating very large orbital floor fracture.*

The eye may also be injured by whatever fractured the orbital floor. Treatment of an orbital fracture is predicated upon a normal eye examination. Treatment of ocular injuries takes precedence over treatment of orbital fractures. Occult globe ruptures, hyphemas and traumatic optic neuropathies should all be treated prior to the orbital fractures.

CT (computed tomography) scanning is the most important test to obtain in evaluating patients with orbital fractures (Fig. 10.2 (b)).[2] Plain orbital X-rays are archaic. CT scans not only allow evaluation of the bony orbit but also allow evaluation of the eye and orbital soft tissues. Appropriate direct coronal views are necessary to delineate and identify properly

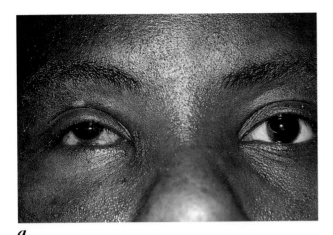

*a*

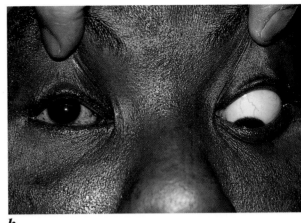

*b*

*c*

**Figure 10.5** *Patient with an orbital fracture presenting with a large right hypertropia in primary gaze (a), loss of downgaze (b), limitation of upgaze (c) secondary to posterior entrapment of the inferior rectus muscle.*

orbital floor fractures. If direct coronal views are impossible to obtain because the patient cannot hyperextend his neck or has an excess of dental fillings, reconstructed axial views will suffice. Various types of orbital fractures can be seen on CT scans. CT scans also allow one to differentiate an orbital fracture from other causes of globe ptosis (Figs 10.3 (a) and (b)). Superior subperiosteal hemorrhages and traumatic encephaloceles secondary to orbital roof fractures may be mistaken for orbital floor fractures. Their treatment is obviously very different. Large fractures may involve the majority of the orbital floor (Figs 10.4 (a) and (b)). If these patients are not enophthalmic at the time of initial evaluation, they will be after the orbital swelling subsides. They will require surgery to correct their enophthalmos.[3] Other patients may have small greenstick-type fractures with obvious entrapment of the inferior rectus or its septae (Figs 10.5 and 10.6). These patients are often initially diplopic, forced ductions are positive, and they often require surgery to obviate their diplopia.

Patients with small fractures and infraorbital paresthesias with numb teeth may not require surgery. This is a very gray area, for infraorbital paresthesias may resolve spontaneously or they may not resolve at all if the infraorbital nerve is severely damaged. On the other hand, if a fragment of bone is impinging upon the infraorbital nerve, the paresthesias may cease after the bone is removed and the nerve decompressed. Delayed onset of infraorbital pain

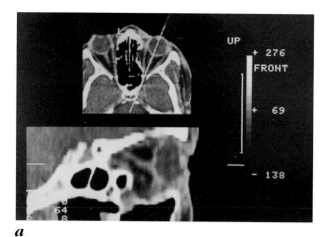
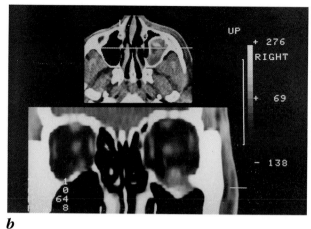

*a*                                                    *b*

**Figure 10.6** *CT scans demonstrating posterior entrapment of the inferior rectus muscle more evident on the sagittal (a) than the coronal scan (b).*

exacerbated by palpation of the inferior orbital rim indicates compression of the infraorbital nerve and is an indication to decompress the infraorbital nerve.[4] Clinical judgment and experience dictate the need for surgery in these patients. Although the past literature has ranged from total therapeutic nihilism ('there is no indication for orbital floor surgery'[5]) to 'the presence of a fracture is an indication for surgery', most now agree that the following are excellent indications for orbital floor fracture repair:[3,6]

1) Diplopia with extraocular muscle entrapment
2) Clinically significant enophthalmos
3) A large fracture evident on computed tomography

## DIPLOPIA WITH EXTRAOCULAR MUSCLE ENTRAPMENT

Patients with orbital floor fractures may have diplopia secondary to muscle injury, orbital hemorrhage, or entrapment of the extraocular muscle or orbital septae in the fracture site. This type of entrapment is most common in patients with small, greenstick-type fractures that trap the muscle. It may also be seen in patients with hinge-type trapdoor floor fractures that have partially reduced themselves, entrapping orbital

contents. The eye may not elevate, may not depress, or may not do either. Clinical examination and CT scanning are usually diagnostic (Fig. 10.5 and 10.6). Conventional wisdom states that these patients should be observed for 7–10 days to see if the diplopia resolves. If the muscle is entrapped, it is not going to resolve without intervention; and prolonged entrapment may result in further loss of muscle function.[7] Muscle entrapment is more the exception than the rule. In the author's experience, motility dysfunction after orbital floor fractures commonly results from entrapment of orbital septae in combination with orbital fat. There is a role for systemic corticosteroids in hastening the resolution of orbital edema if there is a question about entrapment versus a dysfunctional muscle.[8] Systemic corticosteroids hasten the evolution and contract the clinical course of orbital fractures. This may hasten the decision-making process and allow earlier surgery in equivocal cases. If diplopia does not promptly resolve and forced ductions remain positive, surgery is necessary. On the other hand, unnecessary surgery may be avoided by utilizing high-resolution CT scanning and careful evaluation of extraocular motility to differentiate surgically amenable diplopia from diplopia that might well resolve spontaneously.[9] Patients with obvious CT evidence for muscle entrapment, adhesions or enophthalmos benefited from orbital floor fracture repair. Patients with other causes for their diplopia—intramuscular hemorrhage, edema or

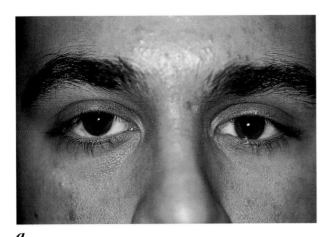
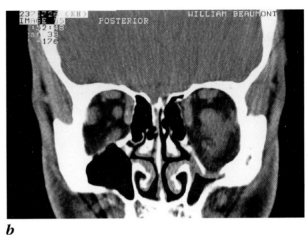

*a*                                              *b*

**Figure 10.7** *Clinically significant and very obvious enophthalmos (a) caused by a large orbital fracture visualized on coronal CT scan (b).*

cranial nerve paresis—did not require surgery. Treating these patients with eye muscle exercises and observation decreased the need for surgery by 50%.[9]

## CLINICALLY SIGNIFICANT ENOPHTHALMOS

Significant enophthalmos, with or without inferior displacement of the globe, is a prima facie indication for repair of an orbital fracture (Fig. 10.7). This clinical presentation results from a very large orbital floor fracture often combined with a fracture of the medial orbital wall. There is little to be gained by waiting several weeks to operate upon these patients. These defects will not resolve without surgical intervention, and it should be accomplished sooner rather than later. Resolution of orbital swelling can be hastened with systemic corticosteroids, if necessary.[8]

Early orbital swelling or hemorrhage may mask the appearance of clinically significant enophthalmos. These patients should be followed closely for the development of enophthalmos, especially if the CT scan demonstrates a significant disruption of the orbital floor (Fig. 10.4 (b)). Systemic corticosteroids (prednisone 80 mg daily) may be used to contract the healing process and detect the development of enophthalmos in a more timely fashion.[8]

## A LARGE FRACTURE ON CT SCAN

This indication is very similar to clinically significant enophthalmos. Patients with large fractures of their orbital floors will very likely develop enophthalmos even if it is not readily apparent immediately after injury (Figs 10.4 and 10.7).[3]

Conventional wisdom states that one should wait 10–14 days after injury before repairing an orbital floor fracture. This is reasonable if a patient has diplopia and entrapment is equivocal. Remember that these rules were made in the pre-CT era, and it is senseless to adhere to them as truth in today's world of excellent imaging studies. A patient with diplopia and obvious entrapment on CT scan (Figs 10.5 and 10.6) should be operated upon as soon as the orbital swelling has subsided, and this can be hastened with the use of systemic corticosteroids. There is nothing to gain by waiting for 10–14 days before releasing an entrapped muscle. Certainly, two weeks of entrapment and ischemia will do little to help the muscle's function.[7]

A patient with obvious enophthalmos and a large fracture on CT should also be operated upon as soon as the orbital edema and hemorrhage have subsided. Early surgery is not as critical in this case because there is no muscle entrapment. A patient with diplopia and no CT evidence for entrapment or adhesions of the extraocular muscles might well be

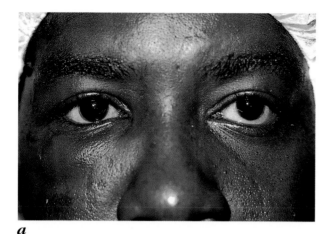

*a*

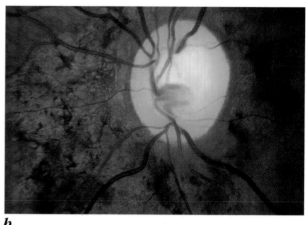

*b*

**Figure 10.8** *Asymmetry of face and flattening of the left malar eminence due to a trimalar fracture. Optic atrophy (b) and a traumatic macular hole (c) undetected prior to surgery.*

*c*

observed for resolution of diplopia.[6,9] In many cases, surgery might be deferred indefinitely.[5,6]

## PATIENT EVALUATION

Evaluation and treatment of any orbital fracture are predicated upon a normal eye examination. A careful ocular examination is necessary to detect concomitant ocular or optic nerve injuries. A blow to the eye and orbit of sufficient force to cause an orbital fracture may also cause any of the ocular injuries described in the section on blunt ocular trauma (Fig. 10.8). Such an injury can also cause a traumatic optic neuropathy that may be exacerbated by orbital surgery. These admonishments are usually heeded by ophthalmologists, but it is amazing how many patients with orbital fractures are taken to the operating room by other

specialities without the benefit of an eye examination. The ophthalmologic disasters that occur could only be pleasing to the plaintiff's bar. There is little, if any, indication to operate upon a patient with an orbital fracture without a complete eye examination. Doing so is violating the standard of care in most communities. Can the author be more clear?

After the eye examination, the whole patient should be looked at (Fig. 10.8). Is the face symmetrical? Are both malar eminences equal, or is one flattened? The lateral and inferior orbital rims should be palpated. Is there discomfort or pain to palpation? This may indicate a concomitant orbital rim or lateral wall fracture that can often be palpated. Can the patient open his mouth without discomfort? This may indicate a trimalar fracture for the masseter and temporalis muscles attach to the zygoma. Whitnall's ligament and the lateral canthal tendon also attach to the zygoma at the lateral orbital wall. Fracture and

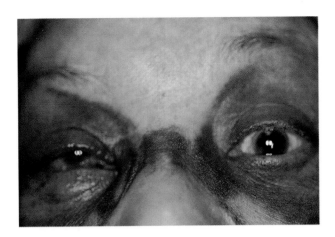

**Figure 10.9** *Periorbital ecchymosis (raccoon eyes) due to basilar skull and orbital roof fractures.*

displacement may cause sagging of the lateral canthus and ptosis of the lateral upper eyelid.

A trimalar fracture is the separation of the zygoma from its attachments to the maxillary, sphenoid, frontal and temporal bones. Usually the zygoma is displaced downward, inward and posteriorly. Orbital floor fractures almost always accompany trimalar fractures and need to be repaired concomitantly. Both can be repaired through a lateral canthotomy and transfornix approach to the orbital floor and lateral wall.

Is there evidence for proptosis, enophthalmos or inferior displacement of the globe? Proptosis is usually not compatible with an orbital floor fracture unless there is extensive swelling and hemorrhage which might mask enophthalmos or a blow-in fracture resulting from the inward displacement of the malar block.[10] Proptosis and downward displacement of the eye should alert the examiner to a superior orbital mass (Fig. 10.3) that might be the result of trauma. Enophthalmos and inferior displacement of the globe are both compatible with an orbital fracture. These can be differentiated by CT scanning, which represents the requisite standard of care in evaluating patients with orbital trauma.

The orbital roof is much thicker than the orbital floor and medial wall. It rarely suffers blowout-type fractures. Orbital roof fractures are almost always accompanied by significant frontal trauma, with or without a superior orbital rim fracture. The patient may present with periorbital ecchymosis (raccoon eyes) (Fig. 10.9) due to orbital roof and basilar skull fractures. Repair, when necessary, is a multidisciplinary affair in company with the ENT (ear, nose and throat) and neurosurgical services.

Extraocular motility should be examined. Do the eyes move freely and conjugately in all directions? An orbital floor fracture may cause an obvious hyper- or

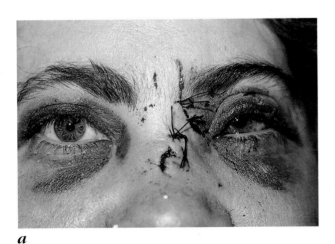

*a*

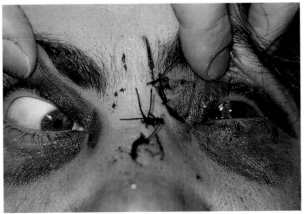

*b*

**Figure 10.10** *Patient with an esotropia in primary gaze (a) with limited abduction of the left eye (b) after periorbital trauma. CT Scanning and forced ductions differentiate a medial orbital wall fracture with entrapment from a sixth-nerve palsy.*

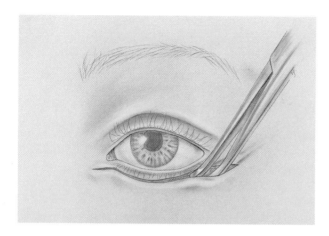

**Figure 10.11** *Subciliary incision to expose the orbital floor should be made as close to the lashes as possible to minimize scarring.*

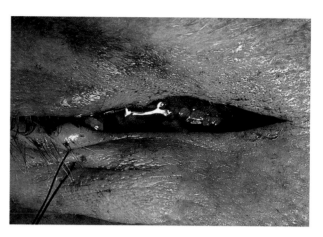

**Figure 10.12** *Extended lateral canthotomy and inferior cantholysis to expose the orbital floor through the fornix.*

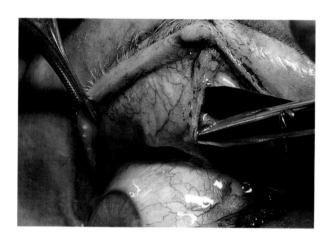

**Figure 10.13** *Surgeon's view: elevating a conjunctival flap to expose the orbital floor through the fornix.*

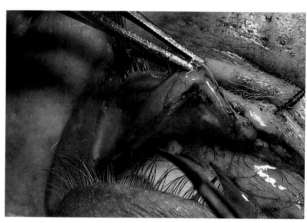

**Figure 10.14** *Surgeon's view: further dissection to expose the inferior orbital rim. The conjunctiva is retracted with sutures and the retractors of the eyelid are grasped with forceps. The plane is between the conjunctiva and retractors and is being dissected with scissors.*

hypotropia with limited elevation or depression of the globe (Figs 10.5 (a)–(c)). Limited horizontal gaze may result from entrapment of the medial rectus by a medial orbital wall fracture (Fig. 10.10). Forced ductions and a CT scan will differentiate this from a sixth-nerve palsy.

The patient should be questioned about pain or numbness over the distribution of the infraorbital nerve. Are the regional teeth numb? Is the sensory deficit improving or worsening?

## ORBITAL FLOOR FRACTURE REPAIR

The orbital floor can be approached transconjunctivally through the fornix or via a transcutaneous

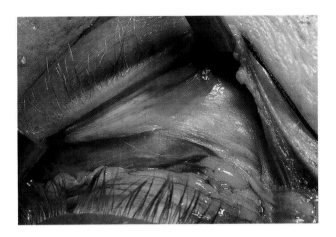

**Figure 10.15** *The eyelid is retracted and the orbital rim is exposed.*

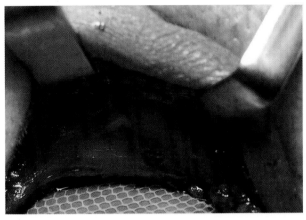

**Figure 10.16** *The orbital rim has been cleaned with gauze, the eyelid is retracted and the globe is protected with a large malleable retractor.*

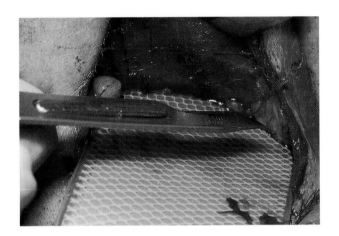

**Figure 10.17** *The periosteum is incised at the inferior orbital rim.*

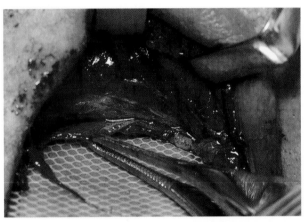

**Figure 10.18** *The periorbita is elevated over the orbital rim. Note the loose adherence of the periosteum to the orbital floor.*

subciliary incision (Fig. 10.11).[11] Direct incision over the orbital rim is archaic, often leaves an unacceptable scar, and should be abandoned. Surgery is performed under general anesthesia. Antecedent infiltration of the incision site and beneath the periosteum with 2% xylocaine containing epinephrine and hyaluronidase facilitates dissection and augments hemostasis. The transconjunctival approach to the orbital floor provides excellent exposure and is cosmetically very acceptable. The author's practice is to augment exposure by performing a canthotomy/cantholysis prior to incising the conjunctiva (Fig. 10.12). The canthotomy incision can be extended over the lateral orbital wall to expose a trimalar fracture (Fig. 10.12). Two 4-0 silk sutures are placed through the eyelid margin and the eyelid is everted. The epinephrine-

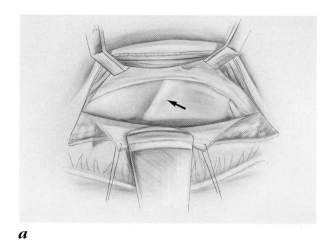

*a*

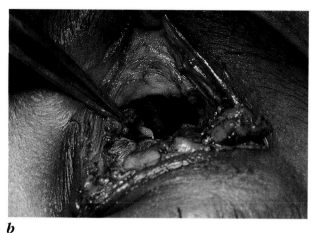

*b*

**Figure 10.19** *Diagram of the orbital floor (arrow indicates position of the infraorbital neurovascular bundle). This position may be very variable. Fractures usually lie medial to the neurovascular bundle (a). The infraorbital neurovascular bundle can be seen in a large orbital floor defect (b).*

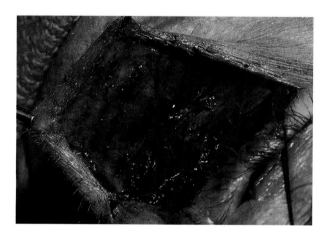

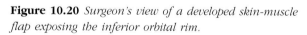

**Figure 10.20** *Surgeon's view of a developed skin-muscle flap exposing the inferior orbital rim.*

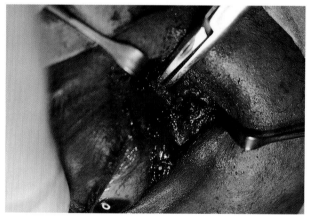

**Figure 10.21** *Reduction of a trimalar fracture by extending a lateral canthotomy incision exposing the lateral orbital wall. Clamp placed behind the lateral orbital wall will be used to elevate and reduce the fracture.*

containing anesthetic solution is infiltrated under the conjunctiva. The conjunctiva is incised with scissors behind the tarsus, and a conjunctival flap is elevated with sharp or cautery dissection (Figs 10.13 and 10.14). The latter is preferred as it allows simultaneous cauterization and dissection. A 6-0 Vicryl suture is placed at the nasal and temporal ends of the incision,

and the conjunctiva is retracted over the globe and clamped to the drapes. The lower eyelid is retracted inferiorly with two Senz (Storz, St Louis, MO) retractors, exposing the inferior orbital rim (Fig. 10.15). The orbital rim is palpated over its entire course and the rim cleaned of overlying tissue with a piece of gauze. With the eyelid retracted inferiorly, the conjunctiva

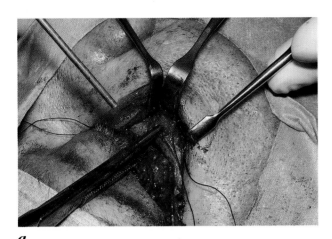

*a*

**Figure 10.22** *Reduction of an inferior orbital rim fracture. The rim is manipulated with a clamp while the malar block fracture is being reduced. The fractured ends are approximated prior to fixation (b).*

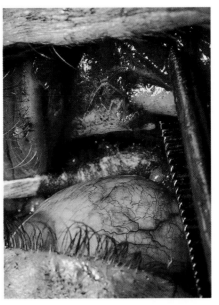

*b*

retracted superiorly and the globe protected with a large malleable retractor (Fig. 10.16), the periorbita over the inferior orbital rim is incised with a 15 blade (Fig. 10.17). Incision is made no more than 2–3 mm from the rim to ensure that the infraorbital nerve is not incised as it exits the infraorbital foramen. The periorbita is dissected from the orbital rim with a Freer elevator. The periorbital is firmly adherent to the orbital rim but is loosely adherent to the orbital floor, and this is very evident when the periorbita is reflected from the orbital rim (Fig. 10.18). A 5-0 Dexon suture is placed through the periorbita and used to retract it superiorly. This exposes the inferior orbital floor (Fig. 10.19).

If a subciliary approach is chosen, an incision is made with a sharp blade just below the cilia of the lower eyelid from the punctum to the lateral canthus (Fig. 10.11). The area has been previously infiltrated with the epinephrine-containing anesthetic solution. The tissue is buttonholed with scissors at the lateral portion of the tarsus, a hemostat introduced and spread. This maneuver separates the lid into a skin-muscle lamella and a septal conjunctival layer (Fig. 10.20). Two 4-0 silk sutures are passed through the eyelid margin, and it is retracted superiorly. The skin-muscle flap is developed to the level of the inferior orbital rim. The flap is retracted with Senz retractors, and the orbital rim is exposed and cleaned with a piece of gauze. Subsequent dissection and exposure utilize the transconjunctival approach.

Exposure of the orbital floor is facilitated by retracting the periorbita superiorly with the 5-0 Dexon suture. A good headlight is necessary to visualize the orbital floor properly. Hemostasis should be obtained with bipolar cautery. Sinus mucosal bleeding is usually easily controlled by packing with neurosurgical cottonoids soaked in Afrin (oxymetazoline HCl 0.05%). Excellent hemostasis should be obtained prior to exploring the orbital floor. Forced ductions should be performed prior to exploring the orbital floor and again after the implant has been placed.

If a trimalar fracture is present, the lateral canthal incision can be extended to expose the lateral orbital wall (Fig. 10.21).[12] The zygomaticofrontal and the zygomaticotemporal fractures may be exposed through this incision. Temporalis muscle may be separated from the lateral orbital wall with a cutting cautery prior to reducing the fracture with a Bristow elevator or an Ochsner clamp (Storz, St Louis, MO) (Fig. 10.21). Either instrument is placed behind the lateral orbital rim and used to elevate and reduce the fracture. The accompanying orbital rim fracture may be reduced simultaneously (Fig. 10.22). After the malar block is reduced, the fracture sites are fixated with miniplates and attention is turned to the orbital floor.[13] If the orbital rim is fractured, there is almost certainly an orbital floor fracture.

Orbital floor fractures typically occur medial to the infraorbital neurovascular bundle and commonly

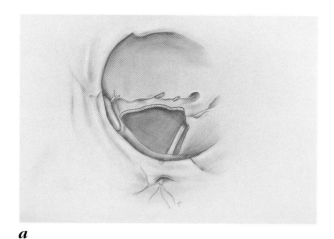
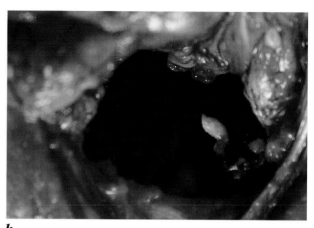

*a*                                                    *b*

**Figure 10.23** *Diagram demonstrating a large orbital floor defect medial to the infraorbital neurovascular bundle (a). Infraorbital neurovascular bundle lying in a large orbital floor defect (b).*

extend medially to involve the medial wall of the orbit. The bone here is thin and easily fractured by compression by the globe or direct trauma to the orbital rim (Fig. 10.23). The lateral aspect of the fracture site is often an intact neurovascular bundle. The orbital floor rarely fractures lateral to the infraorbital neurovascular bundle (Fig. 10.23 (b)). The inferior orbital fissure lies 18–20 mm from the inferior orbital rim. Its periosteal reflections can be mistaken for orbital tissue trapped in a fracture site, and trying to free it can be hemorrhagically embarrassing. Care should be taken lateral to the neurovascular bundle —fractures do not often occur there.

The fracture site has been identified medial to the neurovascular bundle (Fig. 10.24). Identify the infraorbital nerve and the neurovascular bundle. Remember that the nerve is not encased by bone in the posterior orbit—'freeing' the infraorbital nerve while elevating the fracture will sever it, with resultant numbness in the cheek and teeth. Identify the nerve prior to freeing the entrapped orbital contents. The entrapped orbital contents may be elevated from the fracture site using a suction tip and a Freer elevator in a hand-over-hand fashion. The orbital contents are retracted with a malleable retractor. Be careful not to stick this retractor too deep into the orbit or compress the orbital contents with it for too long a period of time. The author suspects that some of the unexplained visual loss after orbital floor surgery is the result of overzealous retraction and failure to

relieve pressure on the orbit at frequent intervals. As the entrapped orbital contents are elevated, they may be isolated with neurosurgical cottonoids. This facilitates elevation. If the orbital contents do not elevate easily, a common occurrence in old fractures, using a Kerrison rongeur to remove some of the bone at the anterior end of the fracture site greatly facilitates elevating the orbital contents from the fracture site. Orbital contents can be freed while working around the fracture site. Intact bone on both sides of the fracture should be identified. The CT scan can be used as a guide to find the posterior extent of the fracture. The back wall of the maxillary sinus lies 10 mm from the orbital apex. If the fracture extends through the solid bone deep to the maxillary sinus, it is probably not reducible without risking potential visual loss. It is better to have some residual diplopia or enophthalmos than to have a blind eye after surgery.

On the other hand, knowing that the posterior wall of the maxillary sinus is 10 mm anterior to the orbital apex allows the surgeon to operate within the maxillary sinus with relative impunity when necessary to reduce a troublesome fracture. This is valuable when trying to reduce a greenstick fracture that has entrapped an extraocular muscle posteriorly (Figs. 10.5 and 10.6). It is also helpful when reducing a very large floor fracture prior to placing a wire mesh implant. A surgeon operating on a variety of orbital floor fractures should be comfortable working in the

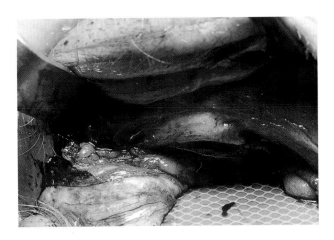

**Figure 10.24** *Orbital floor fracture accompanying an orbital rim fracture.*

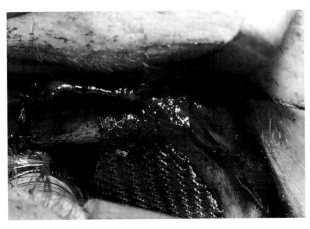

**Figure 10.25** *Prolene mesh implant placed over a small orbital floor defect (shown in Fig. 10.24). A larger defect (Fig. 10.23 (b)) would require either a wire mesh or a rigid Medpore implant to obviate enophthalmos.*

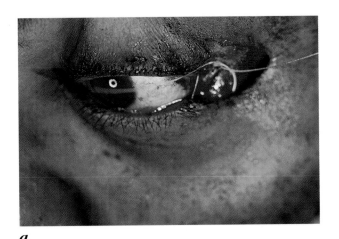

*a*

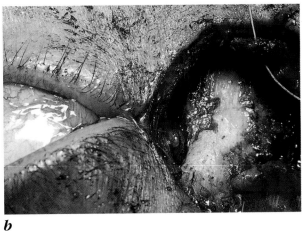

*b*

**Figure 10.26** *The canthus is reapproximated using a 5-0 suture uniting the upper and lower lids and fixating them to the periorbita at the lateral orbital tubercle (b).*

maxillary sinus from above and from the transantral approach.

After reducing the fracture, an implant is placed over the fracture site (Fig. 10.25). Sizing the implant may be facilitated by using X-ray film as a template.[14] The used film is cut to size, slid into the orbit, and outlines the defect to be covered. It is then cut to the proper size and then removed from the orbit to use as a template in sizing the orbital floor implant, be it bone, Medpore or metal. The implant should rest on at least three solid sides of bone around the fracture. The author prefers Medpore implants (Porey

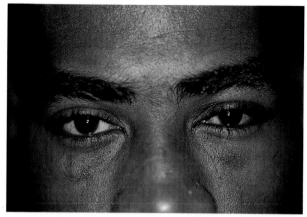

*a*

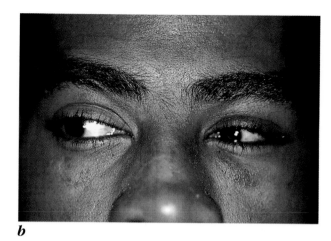

*b*

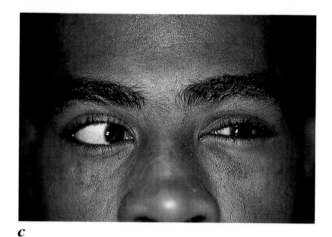

*c*

**Figure 10.27** *Patient with a medial orbital wall fracture and diplopia in lateral gaze due to entrapment of the medial rectus muscle.*

Industries, College Park, GA), usually 1.5 mm thick. Thicker implants (3 mm) are available and quite useful for patients with post-traumatic enophthalmos. Implants are cut to size to cover the fracture site. Large fracture sites may require a wire mesh implant fixated to the back wall of the maxillary sinus and screwed to the inferior orbital rim. If this fails to correct the enophthalmos, orbital volume can be augmented by stacking Medpore plates on the wire mesh implant. Recently, fixation plates have been incorporated into Medpore implants to facilitate fracture repair.

After the fracture has been reduced and the implant positioned, the orbital floor is inspected for hemostasis. Blood oozing from the wound edges needs to be differentiated from mucosal or orbital bleeding. Meticulous hemostasis should be obtained

prior to closure. The periosteum, if intact, is closed with 5-0 Dexon suture. The conjunctiva is recessed with 6-0 Vicryl suture, the canthus reformed with a 5-0 Dexon suture, one arm passed from the upper lid, one from the lower lid, tied, and both arms passed through the periorbita of the lateral orbital wall and tied (Fig. 10.26). After the canthus has been reformed, the wound is closed.

## MEDIAL ORBITAL WALL FRACTURES

The medial wall of the orbit is the thin lamina papyriciae and it is often fractured in conjunction with orbital floor fractures. Isolated medial orbital wall fractures may not require surgical repair. These

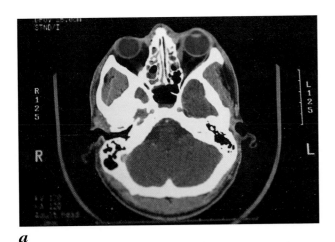

*a*

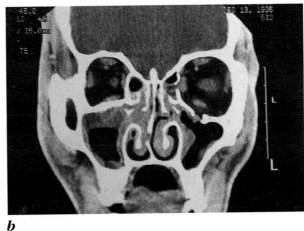

*b*

**Figure 10.28** *CT scan demonstrating medial rectus muscle entrapped in a medial orbital wall fracture.*

patients may present with epistaxis and orbital emphysema after injury to the orbit.[15] Acutely, these patients may be treated with cold compresses, oral antibiotics (cephalexin 500 mg every 6 hours) to prevent infection, and observation.

Rarely, patients with orbital emphysema may have a ball-valve effect.[16] As the patient breathes, air fills the orbit, and a small fracture acts as a one-way valve, letting air enter the orbit from the adjacent ethmoid sinus but not allowing it to exit. Excessive air enters the orbit and causes a compressive optic neuropathy. These patients present with visual loss, an amaurotic or relative afferent pupillary defect, and excessive orbital emphysema. Treatment needs to be emergent and entails enlarging the fracture. A hemostat may be passed along the medial orbital wall through the conjunctiva or through a small skin incision and used to infracture the medial orbital wall. Enlargement of the fracture site, or creation of another fracture, allows the air to egress from the orbit and immediately decompresses the optic nerve. These occurrences are uncommon, but quite dramatic. Immediate recognition and treatment may be sight-saving.

Large medial orbital wall fractures may cause significant enophthalmos and should be repaired.[17] Smaller fractures may cause entrapment of the medial rectus muscle with resultant diplopia (Figs 10.27 and 10.28). These patients may be frankly esotropic in primary gaze and have marked restriction of ocular abduction. They may also be straight in primary gaze and only diplopic in lateral gaze due to their restricted ocular abduction. If diplopia does not promptly resolve (this too can be hastened with a course of corticosteroids), these fractures should be reduced and repaired.

## TECHNIQUE FOR REPAIR OF A MEDIAL ORBITAL WALL FRACTURE

The operative site is infiltrated with the epinephrine-containing anesthetic solution and the nasal mucosa and the ethmoid sinus treated with oxyhydroxazine HC1 0.05% (Afrin) to constrict the mucosa and enhance hemostasis. This is easily accomplished by packing around the endotracheal tube and pouring 60 cc of Afrin into the nostril on the involved side. After 10–15 minutes the mucosa and ethmoid air cells are vasoconstricted and shrunken. Surgery is greatly facilitated.

After the patient is anesthetized, forced ductions are performed by grasping the medial rectus with a forcep and abducting the eye. Forced ductions allow one to determine whether the extraocular muscle is entrapped. They should be repeated after the fracture has been reduced and again after the implant has been placed. A gull-wing incision is then outlined by

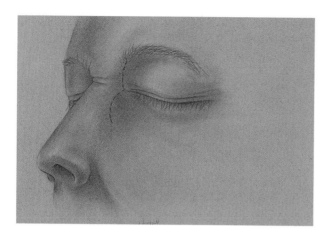

**Figure 10.29** *Gull-wing incision to expose the medial orbital wall.*

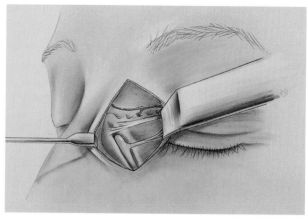

**Figure 10.30** *Diagrammatic representation of the anatomy of the medial orbital wall demonstrating the relationships between the lacrimal sac, medial canthal tendon and the ethmoidal vessels. Fractures are located inferior to the ethmoidal vessels. The medial canthal tendon and the lacrimal sac may be reflected with the periosteum.*

combining a dacrocystorhinostomy (DCR) and a Lynch incision meeting at the medial canthus (Fig. 10.29). The incision is made through the skin and extended to and through the periosteum. Hemostasis is accomplished with cautery. The periosteum is reflected from the underlying bone with a Freer elevator. The lacrimal sac, nasolacrimal duct and medial canthal tendon are elevated from the bone, exposing the underlying medial orbital wall (Fig. 10.30). As with the orbital floor, the periosteum is loosely adherent to the medial orbital wall and elevates easily. A good light source is necessary to inspect the medial orbital wall. The fracture site is usually obvious. The orbital contents may be removed from the fracture site with a malleable retractor and a suction tip or a Freer elevator in a hand-over-hand fashion. Mucosal bleeding may be controlled with the Afrinized cottonoids. The cottonoids may also be used to help reduce the fracture by packing the orbital contents away from the fracture site. After the orbital contents have been reduced, forced ductions are repeated. The eye should abduct freely if the fracture has been totally reduced. If the eye does not move freely, the fracture site should be re-evaluated to make sure that there is not undetected posterior entrapment of the medial rectus. When the eye moves freely, the fracture site is covered with an implant. The author usually uses

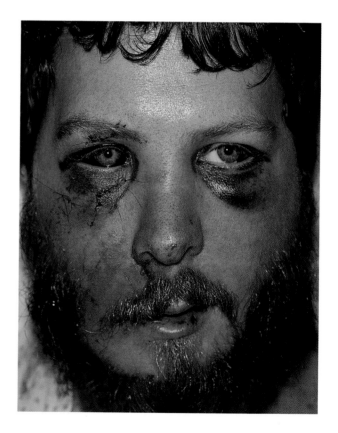

**Figure 10.31** *Traumatic telecanthus due to failure to fixate the severed medial canthal tendon.*

a piece of Medpore, but a metallic mesh implant is equally acceptable. The posterior edge of the implant should be rounded so as not to impale the optic nerve at the orbital apex. If possible, the implant should be placed in a superior–inferior direction to mitigate against the possibility of posterior migration and injury to the optic nerve. If an implant is placed in an anterior–posterior orientation, it should be fixated anteriorly with a screw and plate to prevent posterior migration. Medpore implants with fixation plates incorporated into them are ideal for this technique. After the implant has been placed, the forced ductions should be repeated. The eye should move as freely as it did before the implant was placed. If it does not, repositioning or replacing the implant should be considered.

The surgeon operating in the orbital region should establish the habit of observing the pupil during the course of the operation. Excessive traction or pressure upon the orbital structures may cause pupillary dilatation. Pupillary dilatation may indicate that excessive pressure is being put upon the optic nerve or its blood supply. If detected, this can be corrected before irreparable damage occurs. Pupillary dilatation may also result from pressure upon the ciliary ganglion or short ciliary nerves. This is not as ominous as pressure upon the optic nerve, but the two cannot be differentiated. The pupil should be observed and, if it dilates during surgery, it is necessary to see if it will constrict to normal. This will cause some unneeded aggravation and delays, but will greatly decrease the incidence of visually significant complications from orbital surgery. The practice of suturing the eyelids together prior to orbital surgery is to be eschewed. Those practicing it should really be operating elsewhere. A skilled and experienced orbital surgeon is constantly observing the pupil during the operative procedure. Surgeons who suture the eyelids together during fracture repair are cheating themselves out of the ability to perform forced ductions and to observe the pupil for changes. If the pupil dilates after insertion of the orbital implant, it is an indication that the implant is too large or is putting unacceptable pressure upon orbital structures and should be replaced.

After the implant has been positioned and hemostasis obtained, the periosteum is closed with 5-0 absorbable sutures. This usually repositions the medial canthal tendon if it was removed intact with the periosteum. If the medial canthal tendon was transected, it may be reapproximated to itself with a piece of 5-0 nonabsorbable suture (polypropylene). If there is no medial canthal remnant on the orbital wall, the tendon can be fixated to the orbital wall using a miniplate fixation. A miniplate is screwed to the orbital wall and the medial canthal tendon is fixated (wired or sutured) to the miniplate. Failure to reattach the medial canthal tendon results in a rounding of the canthus and traumatic telecanthus (Fig. 10.31). Subcutaneous tissue is approximated with an absorbable suture and the skin closed.

## COMPLICATIONS OF ORBITAL FRACTURE REPAIR

The most dreaded complication of orbital surgery is immediate postoperative visual loss (Fig. 10.32). Vision should be checked in the recovery room after the patient awakens from anesthesia. Vision may be somewhat blurry due to ointment and discomfort; but visual loss secondary to a compressive or traumatic optic neuropathy or a central retinal artery occlusion is rarely subtle to either the patient or the physician. Optic nerve compression by a hemorrhage or an orbital implant may be relieved by draining the hemorrhage or removing the implant. Treatment is facilitated if compression is detected while the patient is still in the perioperative area. The best treatment is prevention. The orbit should not be closed until meticulous hemostasis has been obtained. Intraoperative hemostasis may be facilitated by the use of bipolar cautery and vasoconstrictors, for example, Afrin and phenylephrine. Postoperative bleeding may occur despite meticulous hemostasis. If a postoperative hemorrhage should occur, no treatment is necessary unless it is causing a compressive optic neuropathy, excessive proptosis, or significant interference with ocular function. Compression may be immediately relieved at the bedside by cutting the canthal sutures and essentially performing a canthotomy and canthalysis as for a traumatic orbital hemorrhage. Most bleeding stops and the canthotomy/ cantholysis may be repaired electively at a later date. Brisk arterial bleeding may require returning to the operating room and identifying and cauterizing the offending vessel. Optic nerve compression by the orbital implant may be detected intraoperatively by observing the pupil. Dilatation of the pupil after insertion of an implant should be sought and, if observed, the implant should be removed and replaced with either a smaller implant or one positioned differently. Usually, removal of an offending implant will result in constriction of the dilated pupil.

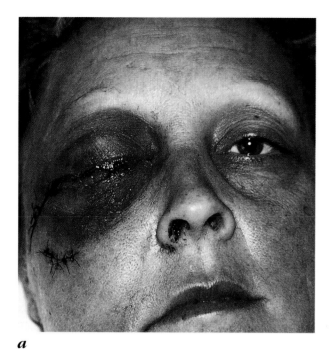

*a*

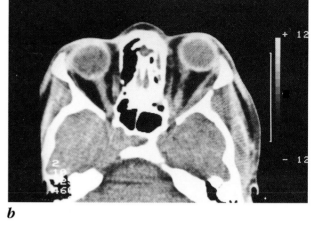

*b*

**Figure 10.32** *Sudden blindness following closed reduction of a trimalar fracture (a). CT scan demonstrates injury to the optic nerve at the orbital apex by a bone fragment (b). Preoperative CT scanning may detect potential complications.*

Occasionally, epinephrine contained in the local anesthetic will partially dilate the pupil. This will be detected if conscious effort is made to examine the pupil continuously during the procedure, not just after inserting an implant. Postoperative pupillary mydriasis may result from extensive manipulation of orbital contents while reducing posterior orbital fractures. This probably results from trauma to the ciliary ganglion.[18] The resultant dilated or tonic pupil is an annoying, but not devastating, complication. It can be managed with dilute cholinergic solutions (pilocarpine 1/10% drops), with or without refractive correction for the defective accommodation. If postoperative visual loss from optic nerve compression is present and there is no obvious orbital hemorrhage, the patient should be returned to the operating room and the implant removed. If the optic nerve compression is due to the implant, visual function may be restored. However, the optic nerve may also be damaged from excessive manipulation and compression during the surgical procedure. Again, prevention is the key to treating these injuries. Excessive traction upon the globe while trying to reduce a fracture may injure the optic nerve. Experienced surgeons are attuned to decreasing their traction upon the globe and examining the pupil at regular intervals during the procedure. Pupillary dilatation is an indication that optic nerve function may be compromised, and traction should be released. The orbit narrows considerably at its apex,

and excessive or misguided manipulation here may damage the optic nerve. Optic nerve injury may be avoided by recognizing that some very posterior fractures are not reducible without excessive risk of injury to the optic nerve. Posterior fractures may be approached through both an orbital incision and a maxillary antrostomy. The posterior wall of the maxillary sinus is approximately 10 mm from the orbital apex. If a fracture extends into the solid bone deep to the posterior wall of the maxillary sinus, it will be difficult to reduce without potential injury to the optic nerve. Fractures anterior to the posterior wall may all be safely reduced by this combined approach. Direct visualization of the fracture in the maxillary sinus avoids blind probing into the deep orbit and potential injury to the optic nerve. Patients with direct injury to the optic nerve or its blood supply will not improve after removal of the implant. The author treats these patients, as well as those with reversible optic nerve compression, with a short course of megadose corticosteroids as for patients with traumatic optic neuropathies. There is no pure scientific evidence that this is beneficial, but results are sometimes impressive; and injured nerves are often helped by prompt treatment with megadose steroids, as demonstrated in the spinal cord injury studies.[19] Methylprednisolone 30 mg/kg is administered as soon as the diagnosis of optic nerve injury is made. Two hours later, 15 mg/kg is infused over 30 minutes; and 15 mg/kg is continued every 6 hours for

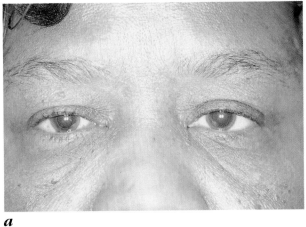

*a*

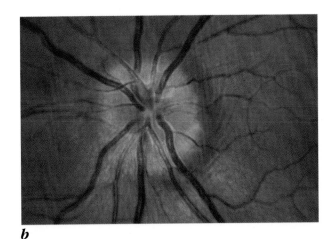

*b*

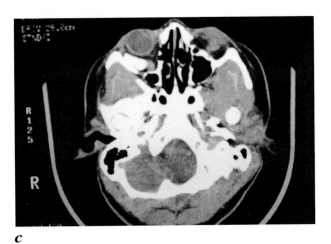

*c*

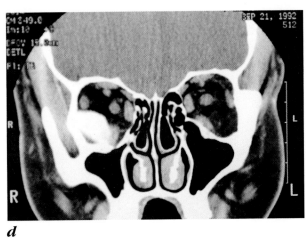

*d*

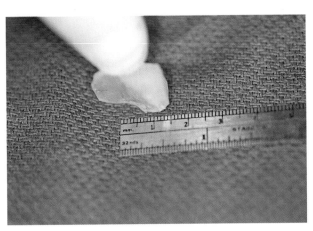

*e*

**Figure 10.33** *Patient presenting with decreased vision in the right eye 4 months after orbital floor fracture repair (a). Right optic disc is swollen, left is normal (b). CT scans demonstrate a large mass in the inferior orbit (c) and (d), which proved to be a large silastic orbital implant (e).*

24–48 hours depending upon the degree of improvement in visual function. Optic nerve compression can occur as a late complication of orbital implants, often because it is not noticed immediately after surgery or the implant migrates postoperatively. Treatment is removal of the implant.

## CASE

A 46-year-old lady (Fig. 10.33 (a)) underwent repair of an orbital floor fracture 4 months prior to evaluation. She presented complaining of decreased vision in the right eye. Visual acuity was 20/25 in the right eye and 20/20 in the left. An obvious afferent pupillary defect was present on the right side. The right optic disc was swollen (Fig. 10.33 (b)); the left was normal. CT scan demonstrated a large mass in the orbital floor thought to be compressing the optic nerve (Fig. 10.33 (c)). A large silastic implant was removed (Fig. 10.33 (d)), disc swelling receded, and visual function normalized.

Other causes of late proptosis following orbital fracture repair include: peri-implant inflammation, sino-orbital fistulas, sinus mucoceles extending into the orbit, and carotid-cavernous fistulas.[20]

An implant that is too thick may cause hyperophthalmia and restriction of extraocular motility (Fig.

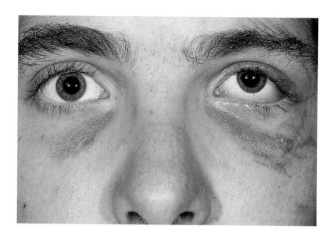

**Figure 10.34** *Hyperophthalmia and restricted motility secondary to an improperly sized silastic implant.*

10.34). Treatment entails removal of the implant and replacing it with one that is more appropriately sized. It is prudent to wait for several weeks for the orbital edema and hemorrhage to subside prior to removal of the implant. Again, systemic corticosteroids may hasten the resolution of orbital edema.

Residual diplopia may occur due to injury to the involved extraocular muscle, orbital hemorrhage and

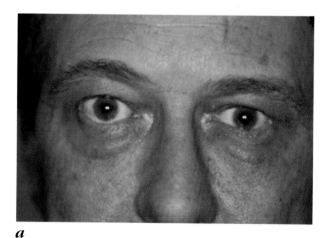

*a*

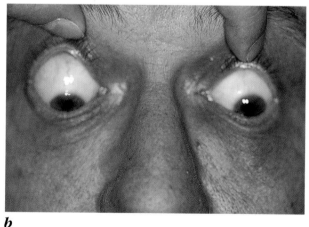

*b*

**Figure 10.35** *Residual vertical diplopia after orbital floor fracture repair (a). There is a small right hypertropia in primary gaze and decreased depression of the right eye (b). Treatment entails a small recession of the left inferior rectus and a posterior fixation suture.*

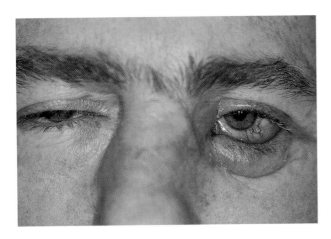

**Figure 10.36** *Lower eyelid malposition due to adherence to orbital bone grafts.*

edema, and failure to free the inferior rectus muscle fully at the time of surgery. The latter will not occur if the surgeon visualizes the posterior extent of the fracture, performs forced ductions before, during and after surgery, and enters the maxillary sinus to free the muscle from below if he or she cannot visualize that it was freed from above. If certain that the muscle was freed from the fracture site during the procedure, the patient may be observed over a 6-month period for resolution of diplopia. If there is any doubt that the muscle entrapment was relieved at surgery, a high-resolution coronal CT scan of the orbit may resolve the issue. If there is no evidence for muscle or septal

entrapment on a high-quality CT scan, the patient should be observed. Diplopia may be obviated by patching or, if the deviation is not too great, a press-on Fresnel prism (3M Healthcare, MN). If diplopia does not resolve after 6 months, it may be improved with eye muscle surgery. Large recessions of both the superior and inferior recti of the involved eye[21] have been shown to increase the range of binocularity. It may be necessary to perform eye muscle surgery on the uninvolved eye. A small resection or recession of the uninjured inferior rectus accompanied by a posterior fixation suture (Faden procedure) may align the eyes in primary gaze and increase the range of fusion in downgaze by hindering the motion of the uninjured eye in downgaze (Fig. 10.35).

Eyelid malpositions occur due to scarring of the eyelid or adherence of the eyelid to the inferior orbital rim (Fig. 10.36). Eyelids are especially prone to adhering to exposed bone grafts. Treatment is lysis of the adhesions and vertical lengthening of the eyelid with a posterior lamella graft of hard palate, tarsoconjunctiva or ear cartilage. Refractory cases may require removal of some of the implanted material and covering of the orbital rim with viable tissue. A periosteal-temporalis fascia flap combined with a hard-palate or ear-cartilage graft can be very useful in refractory cases.

Traumatic telecanthus (Fig. 10.31) occurs when the medial canthal tendon is not reattached after it has been severed or after the bone it attaches to has been fractured and not properly fixated. Treatment in the past entailed transnasal wiring to tighten and fixate the canthus, but the miniplate revolution and widespread acceptance of rigid fixation techniques have made transnasal wiring all but obsolete.

## REFERENCES

1  Smith B, Regan WF Jr. Blow-out fracture of the orbit: mechanism and correction of internal orbital fracture. *Am J Ophthalmol* 1957; **44**: 733.

2  Grove AS. Computed tomography in the management of orbital trauma. *Ophthalmology* 1982; **89**: 433–40.

3  Hawes MJ, Dortzbach RK. Surgery on orbital floor fractures. Influence of time of repair and fracture size. *Ophthalmology* 1983; **90**: 1066–70.

4  Boush GA, Lemke BN. Progressive infraorbital nerve hypesthesia as a primary indication for blow-out fracture repair. *Ophthalmic Plastic Reconstr Surg* 1994; **10**: 206.

5  Putterman AM, Stevens T, Urist MJ. Nonsurgical management of blowout fractures of the orbital floor. *Am J Ophthalmol* 1974; **77**: 232–9.

6  Dutton JJ. Management of blow-out fractures of the orbit. *Surv Ophthalmol* 1991; **35**: 279–80.

7  Smith B, Lisman RD, Simonton J, Della Rocca R. Volkmann's contracture of the extraocular muscles following blowout fracture. *Plastic Reconstr Surg* 1984; **74**: 200–16.

8  Millman AL, Della Rocca R, Spector S, Leibeskind AL, Messina A. Steroids and orbital blowout fractures—a new systematic concept in medical management and surgical decision-making. *Adv Ophthalmol Plastic Reconstr Surg* 1987; **6**: 291–300.

9  Everhard J, Halm YS, Koorneef L, Zonneveld FW. Conservative therapy frequently indicated in blow-out fractures of the orbit. *Med Tijdscher Geneeskd* 1991; **135**: 1226–8.

10 Raflo GT. Blow-in and blow-out fractures of the orbit: clinical correlations and proposed mechanisms. *Ophthalmic Surg* 1984; **15**: 114–19.

11 McCord CD, Moses JL. Exposure of the inferior orbit with fornix incision and lateral canthotomy. *Ophthalmic Surg* 1979; **10**: 53–63.

12 Nunery WR. Lateral canthal approach to repair of trimalar fractures of the zygoma. *Ophthalmic Plastic Reconstr Surg* 1985; **1**: 175–83.

13 Wesley RE. Current techniques for repair of complex orbital fractures. Miniplate fixation and cranial bone grafts. *Ophthalmology* 1992; **99**: 1766–72.

14 Allen CS, Shin JW, Westfall CT. Simplified method of sizing orbital implants. *Am J Ophthalmol* 1995; **120**: 260–1.

15 Zimmer-Galler JE, Bartley GB. Orbital emphysema—case reports and a review of the literature. *Mayo Clin Proc* 1994; **69**: 115–21.

16 Fleishman JA, Beck RW, Hoffman RO. Orbital emphysema as an ophthalmologic emergency. *Ophthalmology* 1984; **91**: 1389–91.

17 Leone CR, Lloyd WC, Rylander G. Surgical repair of medial wall fractures. *Am J Ophthalmol* 1984; **97**: 349–56.

18 Bodker FS, Cytryn AS, Putterman AM et al. Post-operative mydriasis after repair of orbital floor fracture. *Am J Ophthalmol* 1993; **115**: 372–5.

19 Bracken MB, Shepard MJ, Collins WF et al. Methylprednisolone or naloxone treatment after acute spinal cord injury: 1 year follow-up data. *J Neurosurg* 1992; **76**: 23–31.

20 Stewart MG, Patrinely AP, Appling WD, Jordan DR. Late proptosis following orbital floor fracture repair. *Arch Otolaryngol Head Neck Surg* 1995; **121**: 649–52.

21 Kushner BJ. Paresis and restriction of the inferior rectus muscle after orbital floor fracture. *Am J Ophthalmol* 1982; **94**: 81–6.

# Chapter 11 Management of traumatic optic neuropathy

*Thomas C Spoor and John McHenry*

## INTRODUCTION

Visual loss caused by trauma to the optic nerve is a well recognized sequela to craniofacial trauma. This chapter discusses the differential diagnosis, and medical and surgical treatment of pure and complex optic nerve injuries.

Some optic nerve injuries are obvious and treatable if detected early, and the visual loss may be totally reversible. Other injuries are more subtle and may only be detected after a careful ophthalmologic examination. Visual loss may be mild or total. These injuries may be divided into complex traumatic optic neuropathies—those associated with obvious cranio-orbital injury—and pure traumatic optic neuropathies resulting from indirect trauma to the optic nerve.

Traumatic injuries to the optic nerve may be obvious—total, sudden loss of vision, or subtle—decreased visual acuity and a visual field defect. Some traumatic optic neuropathies are untreatable. There is no successful treatment for complete transection or avulsion of the optic nerve (Fig. 11.1). Anterior transection of the optic nerve is usually accompanied by a very obvious fundus appearance of hemorrhage and infarction (Fig. 11.2). A more posterior transection (Fig. 11.3) will initially manifest a normal-appearing optic nerve and retina. The only objective evidence for visual dysfunction may be the presence of an afferent pupillary defect. These injuries are easy to diagnose by detecting the presence of an afferent pupillary defect (Fig. 11.4) or an inverse afferent pupillary defect if the involved pupil is dilated (Fig. 11.5). The relative afferent

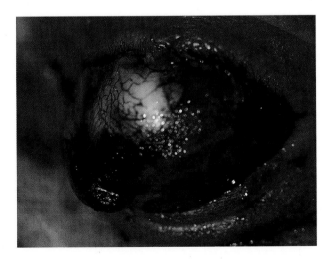

**Figure 11.1 (a)** *Avulsion of the left optic nerve resulting from an altercation.*

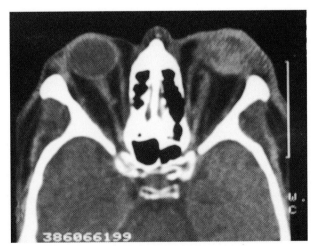

**Figure 11.1 (b)** *CT scan demonstrating avulsion of the optic nerve. Also note the disruption of ocular contents evident in this scan.*

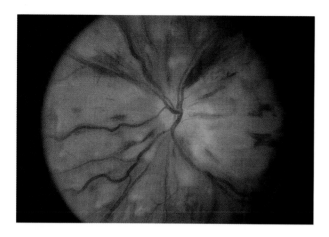

**Figure 11.2** *Hemorrhage and infarction of the retina after anterior avulsion of the optic nerve.*

normal immediately after a severe traumatic injury to the optic nerve. If the optic nerve is injured immediately behind the eye (Fig. 11.1), the blood supply to the posterior globe and optic nerve will be disrupted, and the fundus will appear obviously abnormal (Fig. 11.2). A more posterior injury to the optic nerve may totally disrupt visual function, but the optic disc will appear totally normal (Fig. 11.3 (a)). After four to six weeks, optic atrophy will ensue as the retinal ganglion cells die as a result of descending optic atrophy (Fig. 11.3 (b)). Injury to the cell's axon results in the subsequent death of its cell body, the retinal ganglion cell. To reiterate, detection of an afferent pupillary defect is the key to diagnosing traumatic optic neuropathies.

pupillary defect is the *sine qua non* of an optic nerve injury, but detectable only if it is looked for. It should be remembered that even with total visual loss in one eye due to optic nerve dysfunction, under equal illumination pupils will appear equally sized and normal (Fig. 11.4 (a)). It is important to remember that the optic disc may appear perfectly

## INCIDENCE

Traumatic optic neuropathies are more common than is appreciated in the literature.[1-4] The author's team examined a series of consecutive patients admitted to the cranial trauma unit at Detroit Receiving Hospital, excluding those patients dying within 24 hours of injury, and detected a 15% incidence of traumatic optic neuropathy detected by a totally objective pupillary examination.[5] This is much greater than the 2–3% incidence that had been previously described.[3,4]

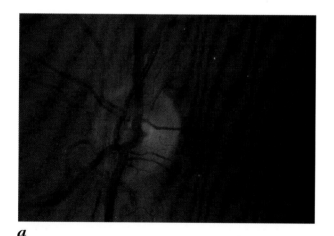

*a*

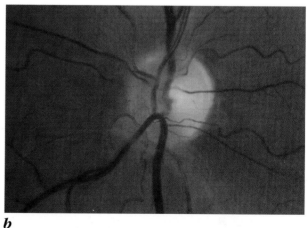

*b*

**Figure 11.3** *(a) Normal-appearing optic nerve and retina in a totally blind eye whose optic nerve was skewered by a ski pole. (b) Obvious atrophy of the optic nerve six weeks after injury due to descending degeneration.*

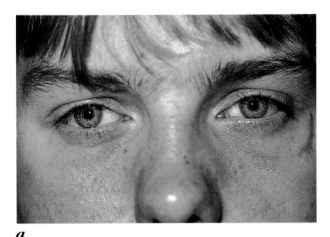
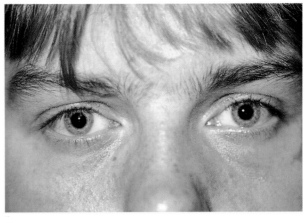

*a*                                                                              *b*

**Figure 11.4** *Relative afferent pupillary defect. Light is directed into the normally sighted eye, and both pupils constrict briskly. As light is directed into the eye with the optic neuropathy, both pupils paradoxically dilate.*

## MANAGEMENT

Detection is the key to management of traumatic optic neuropathies. Awareness that this entity exists and may be subtle is an excellent beginning. Realization that some forms of traumatic optic neuropathy are eminently treatable is also important. These patients often have concomitant cranio-orbital trauma with orbital hemorrhage or a periorbital subperiosteal hemorrhage compressing their optic nerves and elevating the intraocular pressure (Fig. 11.6). Sufficiently high intraocular pressure may result in a central retinal artery occlusion and irreparable

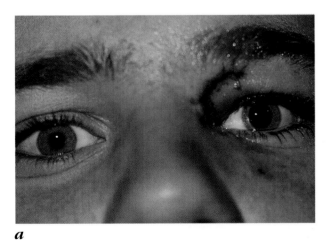
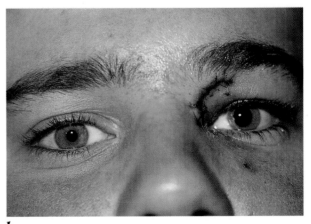

*a*                                                                              *b*

**Figure 11.5** *Inverse relative afferent pupillary defect. Orbital injury has dilated the left pupil as well as injured the optic nerve. As the light is directed into the left pupil, the normal right pupil paradoxically dilates. When the light is directed into the normal right pupil it briskly constricts. The left pupil remains dilated due to the afferent injury.*

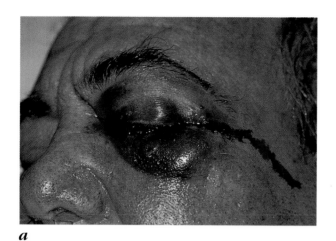

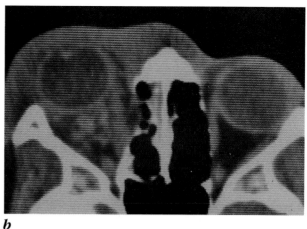

*a*

*b*

**Figure 11.6** *Severe orbital hemorrhage elevating intraocular pressure and causing a compressive (and readily reversible) traumatic optic neuropathy (a). CT scan demonstrating diffuse orbital hemorrhage (b).*

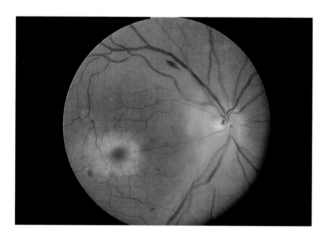

**Figure 11.7** *Central retinal artery occlusion secondary to elevated intraorbital pressure.*

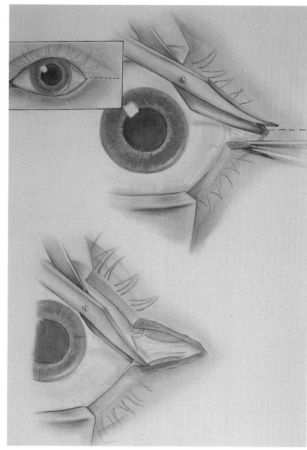

visual loss (Fig. 11.7). Immediate lateral canthotomy/cantholysis relieves optic nerve compression and intraocular pressure elevation resulting from an orbital hemorrhage and may dramatically restore visual function. This should be accomplished expeditiously and may be performed in the emergency room with a local anesthetic by any physician comfortable with the anatomy of this region.

**Figure 11.8** *Technique of canthotomy and cantholysis.*

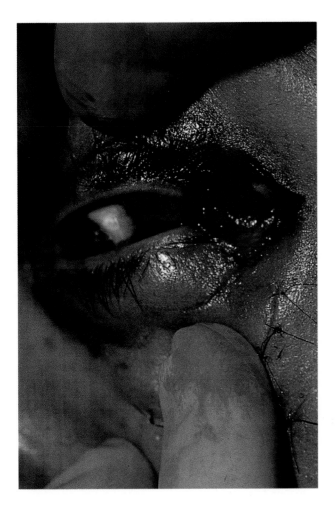

**Figure 11.9** *Appearance of eyelids after an adequate cantbotomy/cantholysis.*

After local anesthetic has been infiltrated into the region, the canthus is clamped with a hemostat and incised with scissors. This is the canthotomy portion of the procedure and is in itself inadequate to decompress an orbital hemorrhage. A cantholysis must be performed. This is accomplished by grasping the lower lid with a forcep and stretching it outward until you can feel the attachments of the lid to the orbital rim. These attachments are then lysed with scissors, and orbital pressure is usually relieved (Fig. 11.8). If further decompression is necessary, the upper eyelid may be treated in a similar fashion (Fig. 11.9). The canthotomy/cantholysis must be performed completely in order to decompress an orbital hemorrhage. After the hemorrhage has resolved, the canthus can easily be repaired under local anesthetic

by suturing the severed upper and lower lids together to approximate the canthal angle and then suturing both to the periorbita inside the orbital rim at the level of the lateral orbital tubercle to reapproximate the eyelids in proper apposition to the globe.

Techniques have been described to decompress the floor of the orbit emergently with a hemostat;[6] but in the author's experience this is rarely necessary if an adequate canthotomy/cantholysis has been performed. If loculated and well demarcated, orbital hemorrhages may be localized by computed tomography and/or ultrasonography and drained with a 22-gauge needle (Fig. 11.10 (a)–(c)).

If visual loss after an orbital hemorrhage has been severe or prolonged, the author routinely treats the patients with a bolus of intravenous methylprednisolone, 30 mg/kg, and continues 15 mg/kg every six hours for 48 hours.[7]

Subperiosteal orbital hemorrhages (Fig. 11.11) are much less common than orbital hemorrhages and often resolve spontaneously[8] but may acutely compromise visual function by compressing the optic nerve. When this occurs, they may be easily evacuated from the subperiosteal space by incising through skin and periosteum and elevating the periosteum from the orbital rim. The hemorrhage is then immediately encountered and may be evacuated with suction (Fig. 11.11 (c)). Bone bleeding may be controlled with bone wax and the incision closed.

In a rare type of orbital hemorrhage, bleeding is confined to the optic nerve sheath. Compression of the optic nerve by this localized hemorrhage causes decreased vision often accompanied by the fundus appearance of a central retinal vein occlusion (Figs. 11.12 (a)–(c)). CT scan demonstrates enlargement of the optic nerve sheath. Drainage of hemorrhage by expeditious optic nerve sheath decompression may restore visual function.[9] Most traumatic optic neuropathies (TONs) do not have an easily discernible and treatable etiology. These may occur in conjunction with other craniofacial injuries (complex) or may occur after isolated periorbital trauma, sometimes almost trivial trauma. The site of injury in these patients is the optic canal, through which the optic nerve traverses between brain and orbit (Fig. 11.13). Injury to the optic nerve may be primary or secondary. Primary injuries include avulsion and transection of the optic nerve or interruption of its blood supply, resulting in infarction of neural tissue. Direct injury and disruption of optic nerve axons may be caused by gunshot wounds, knife wounds and bone fragments from displaced fractures of the optic canal and orbit.

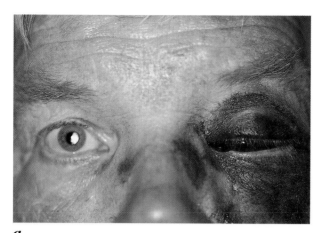

*a*

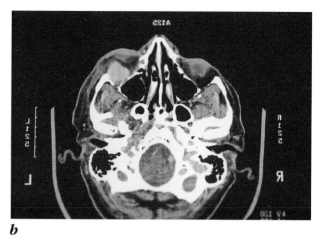

*b*

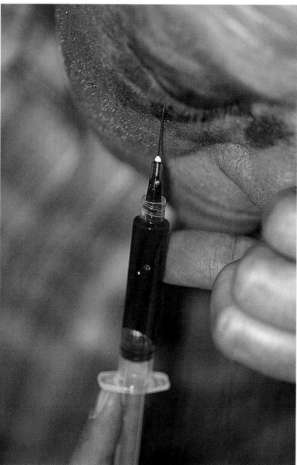

*c*

**Figure 11.10** *Patient with an orbital hemorrhage (a), localized on CT scan (b), and drained by fine-needle aspiration (c).*

Indirect injury to the optic nerve, the classic pure traumatic optic neuropathy, may result from acceleration/deceleration injuries of the globe resulting in stretching, tearing, torsion or contusion of the optic nerve and its blood supply tethered in the optic canal (Fig. 11.14).

Skeletal deformation transmitted to the optic canal from adjacent bony structures may cause compression, ischemia, and devascularization of the optic nerve (Fig. 11.15). Secondary injury occurs at both a subcellular level and a macroscopic level. These secondary events are what the author and colleagues believe we are treating with corticosteroids and extracranial optic canal decompression.

Immediately after primary injury to the optic nerve, biochemical changes begin to occur that may result in further destruction of adjacent axons. These changes affect the microcirculation of the axon, lipid peroxidation, and lysosomal and membrane stabilization. The response of optic nerve tissue to primary injury is activation of a cascade of biochemical reactions which exacerbates the damage caused by the primary injury. These reactions preclude free radicals causing lipid peroxidation and further tissue destruction. Lipid peroxidation produces progressive, delayed, neurologic damage to the optic nerve several hours after injury. This is exacerbated by a decrease in blood flow secondary to intravascular coagulation and vasoconstriction.[10]

These changes may be positively affected by the early use of megadose corticosteroids. Methylprednisolone is thought to prevent lipid peroxidation

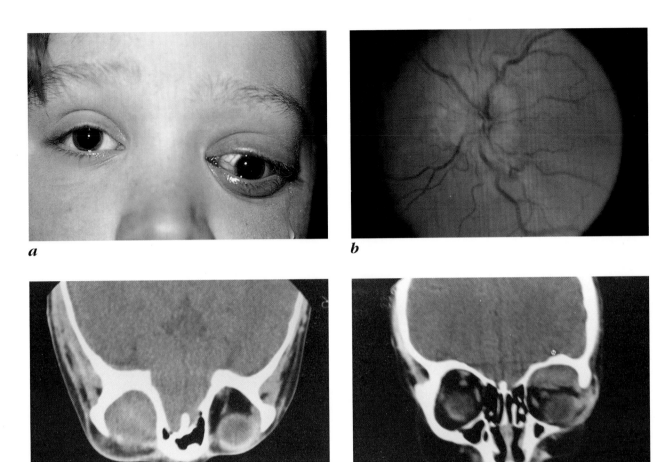

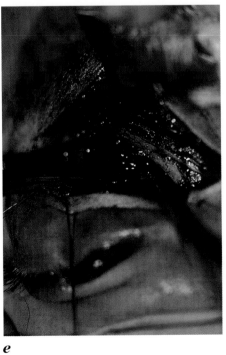

**Figure 11.11** *Child with a subperiosteal orbital hemorrhage (a), decreased vision and a swollen optic disc (b) after an automobile accident. CT scans demonstrate large superior subperiosteal hemorrhage ((c) axial, (d) coronal). Subperiosteal hemorrhage evacuated surgically (e).*

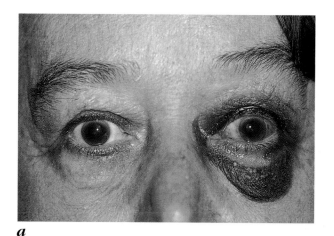

*a*

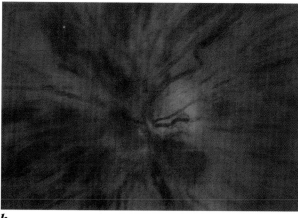

*b*

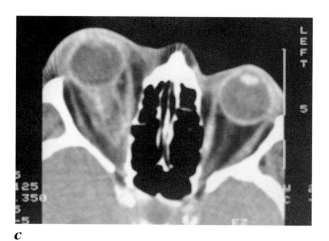

*c*

**Figure 11.12** *Lady struck in the left eye with a fist and noted rapidly decreased vision in the left eye (a). Fundus appearance of venous stasis retinopathy not compatible with no light perception vision (b). CT scan demonstrating optic nerve sheath hemorrhage (c). Visual function improved markedly after emergent optic nerve sheath decompression.*

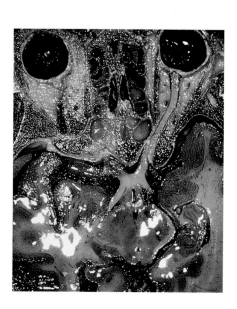

**Figure 11.13** *Axial cadaver section demonstrating the course of the optic nerve extending from the eye to the brain through the optic canal.*

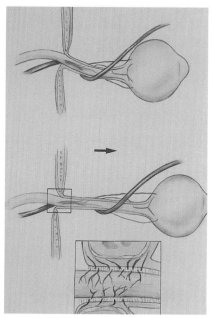

**Figure 11.14** *Acceleration/deceleration injury to the optic nerve secondary to stretching the optic nerve in the optic canal and avulsing the pial vessels.*

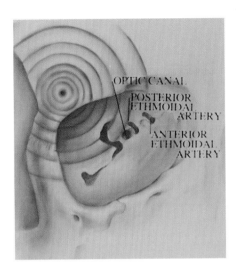

**Figure 11.15** *Skeletal deformation can be caused by pressure waves extending to the optic canal from adjacent bone.*

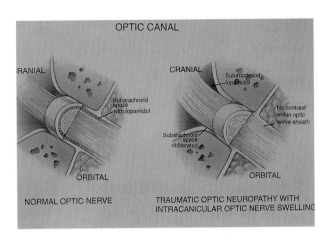

**Figure 11.16** *Cerebrospinal fluid normally flows from the brain to the intraorbital optic nerve through the optic canal (a). Swelling of the traumatized optic nerve compresses it against the bony walls of the optic canal thus further compromising visual function (b).*

and interrupt this cascade of secondary neurologic damage at the biochemical level.[10] As with spinal cord injuries, a comparable but not totally scientific analogy, treatment within the first 8 hours after injury seems to have a beneficial effect.[11,12] In the author's experience, patients receiving megadose corticosteroids within 8 hours of injury had a better visual outcome than those patients receiving steroids more than 8 hours after injury. It is best to administer megadose corticosteroids as soon after injury as feasible. When possible these are administered in the emergency room as soon as the diagnosis of traumatic optic neuropathy is made. It is suggested that referring physicians start administering intravenous steroids prior to transporting the patient to hospital.

When administered more than 8 hours after injury, megadose corticosteroids exert a glucocorticoid effect, it is believed by reducing edema and secondary compression of the axons in the optic canal (Fig. 11.16). Relief of compression allows viable axons to regain function with resultant improvement in visual function.

As soon as possible after diagnosing a traumatic optic neuropathy, an intravenous bolus of methylprednisolone, 30 mg/kg over a 30-minute period is administered.[12] Slow administration over a 30-minute period is necessary to minimize potential cardiac arrhythmias. Two hours later, due to the short serum half-life of methylprednisolone, another bolus of

15 mg/kg is administered. Methylprednisolone is continued at 15 mg/kg every 6 hours for 48 hours. If visual function has improved significantly, steroids are rapidly tapered to 80 mg oral prednisone for 3 days, decreased to 60 mg prednisone for 3 days, 40 mg prednisone for 3 days and finally 20 mg prednisone for 3 days. In the author's experience, all patients with initial visual acuity of 20/100 or better improved on this regimen. Patients with visual acuity of 20/200 or worse (legal blindness) may or may not show improvement. Those patients not improving on the intravenous steroid regimen and those who demonstrate initial improvement and later deterioration in visual function as the steroids are tapered are offered extracranial optic canal decompression.[13,14] Extracranial optic canal decompression (ECOCD) relieves compression of the optic nerve in the optic canal that may not have been relieved by intravenous megadose steroids.

## EXTRACRANIAL TRANSETHMOIDAL OPTIC CANAL DECOMPRESSION

Extracranial optic canal decompression may be performed through the nose, through the maxillary antrum, or through an external ethmoidectomy. It may be performed with an endoscope or with direct

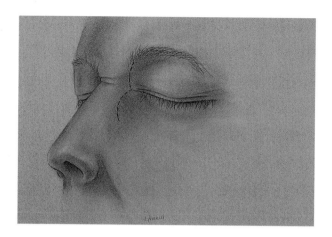

**Figure 11.17** *Skin incision outlined for extracranial optic canal decompression via an external ethmoidectomy.*

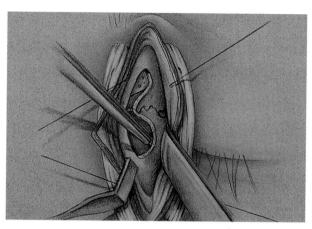

**Figure 11.18** *Cotton bolsters are used to enhance exposure and hemostasis, facilitating extracranial optic canal decompression.*

visualization. Each technique has its sometimes vocal advocates. The author prefers an external ethmoidectomy and microsurgical removal of the medial wall of the optic canal with binocular visualization and illumination with the operating microscope. This can be accomplished transcutaneously by combining a Lynch and a dacryocystorhinostomy incision meeting at the medial canthus (Fig. 11.17) or transconjunctivally, avoiding an external incision but sacrificing some exposure. The exposure obtained through the transcutaneous incision is preferable. Prior to surgery, the medial canthal region is infiltrated with local anaesthetic with epinephrine. The author uses an equal mixture of 2% xylocaine with 1:100 000 epinephrine, 0.75% bupivacaine with 1:100 000 epinephrine with 1 cc of hyaluronidase per 10 cc of anesthetic solution. The resultant vasoconstriction enhances hemostasis, and the anesthetic provides postoperative pain relief. Twenty to thirty cc of oxymetazoline HC1 0.05% (Afrin, Scherring-Plough, Memphis, TN) is instilled into the nose on the involved side. Gauze packing around the endotracheal tube keeps the majority of the solution in the nose and ethmoid sinus and prevents it from draining into the hypopharynx. Afrinization of the ethmoid sinus and nasal mucosa 15 minutes prior to surgery enhances hemostasis and greatly facilitates surgery.

A gull-wing incision is made, cutting directly to the periosteum. Hemostasis is obtained with cautery, and cotton bolsters are sutured to the edges of the

incision further to enhance hemostasis and exposure (Fig. 11.18). The periosteum is incised and reflected from bone with a Freer elevator. The lacrimal sac and the nasolacrimal duct are elevated and reflected laterally. If damaged, a dacryocystorhinostomy may be performed at the conclusion of the procedure. The medial canthal tendon may also be reflected with the periosteum. Periosteum is reflected to the level of the trochlea, exposing the medial orbital wall.

The medial wall of the orbit may be fractured into the ethmoid sinus with a hemostat, or a front sinusotomy may be performed with a drill. The bone in the fronto-ethmoid region is removed piecemeal with a Kerrison rongeur (Stortz Instruments, St Louis, MO) (Fig. 11.19). The ethmoid sinus mucosa is extirpated with Takahashi (Stortz Instruments, St Louis, MO) forceps. Bleeding is usually minimal due to the antecedent Afrinization of the nasal and ethmoid sinus mucosa. The medial wall of the orbit may now be removed with Takahashi forceps (Fig. 11.19). The periorbita should be left intact. The key to safely performing this operation is to keep the periorbita intact and protected with a malleable retractor. This prevents inadvertent injury to the orbital contents. After removal of the medial orbital wall and the ethmoid sinus mucosa, the anterior wall of the sphenoid sinus is exposed. Hemostasis is obtained if necessary with Afrinized cottonoids. While hemostasis is being obtained over the sphenoid sinus, the lateral nasal mucosa is injected with epinephrine

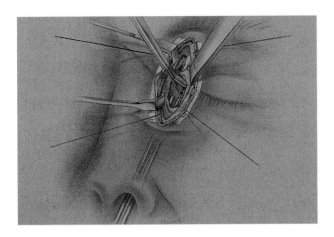

**Figure 11.19** *Removal of the medial orbital wall and ethmoidal air cells.*

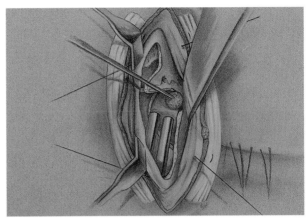

**Figure 11.20** *The medial wall of the optic canal is thinned with a diamond burr passed through the incision. The operative field is constantly irrigated with an irrigating/aspirating cannula passed through the nose.*

containing anesthetic solution. Enough mucosa is excised to allow entry into the ethmoid and sphenoid sinus with a double-barrel irrigating and aspirating cannula. The irrigating/aspirating suction allows subsequent drilling to be done under a constant stream of irrigating saline. This allows removal of the medial wall of the optic canal without the generation of excessive heat, which could damage the optic nerve (Fig. 11.20). The middle turbinate may have been removed prior to this time to obtain adequate exposure.

At this point, hemostasis has been obtained, and the anterior wall of the sphenoid sinus is accessible from both the original incision and the nose. For the surgeon unfamiliar with the ethmoid and sphenoid sinus anatomy, initial entries into the sphenoid sinus may be anxious moments. Is this truly the anterior wall? Could this be the posterior wall, and am I about to enter the brain? Where is the carotid artery?

Enter the sphenoid sinus inferomedially utilizing a small curette or elevator. The anterior wall may then be removed with a small Kerrison or a sphenoid sinus rongeur. The sphenoid sinus mucosa may be removed with Takahashi forceps and hemostasis obtained with an Afrinized cottonoid. This anatomy may be very much deranged in a patient with severe mid-face trauma. Profuse bleeding or CSF leaks may be encountered at this juncture.

The lateral wall of the sphenoid sinus is the medial wall of the optic canal. The anterior portion of this bone needs to be removed in order to decompress the intracanalicular optic nerve. A very helpful landmark is the confluence of periorbital fibers at the orbital apex (Fig. 11.21). This appears whiter than the surrounding periorbita and is a reliable anatomic landmark of the orbital apex. After the orbital apex is identified by the confluence of fibers, the medial wall of the optic canal is removed. The bone may already be fractured, in which case elevating it from the optic nerve ends the operation quickly. Fractures here are relatively uncommon. The bone is usually thick and needs to be thinned with a microdrill and diamond burr (Fig. 11.20) and removed with a curette (Fig. 11.22). Drilling the optic canal must be done under a constant stream of irrigation. The author uses an irrigating/aspirating suction device, entering the surgical field through the nose and resting on the back wall of the sphenoid sinus (Fig. 11.21). Constant irrigation prevents damage to the underlying optic nerve fibers from heat generated by drilling. As the bone is sufficiently thinned, it can be elevated from the underlying optic nerve with a microcurette. A stapedial rongeur and Montgomery picks and elevators (Stortz Instruments, St Louis, MO) are useful in this dissection. Drilling should proceed superiorly and medially. Drilling inferior to the annulus should be avoided, for inadvertent injury to the carotid artery may result in uncontrollable hemorrhage. Inadvertent injury to the dura superiorly may result in a CSF leak that can easily be repaired at the conclusion of the

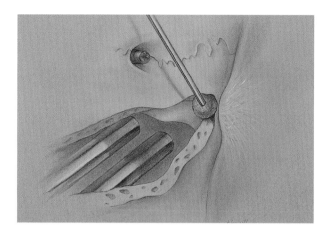

**Figure 11.21** *The confluence of periosteal fibers appears white, identifying the apex of the orbit and the annulus of Zinn. The medial orbital wall and optic canal are being thinned with a microdrill under constant irrigation.*

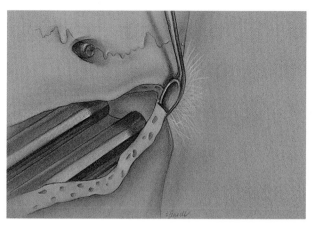

**Figure 11.22** *The thinned medial wall of the optic canal is removed with a microcurette.*

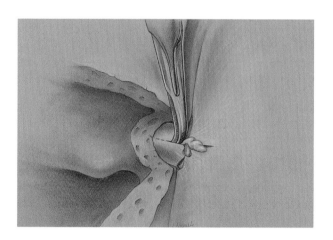

**Figure 11.23** *Incision of the orbital apex and optic nerve dura at the conclusion of the procedure.*

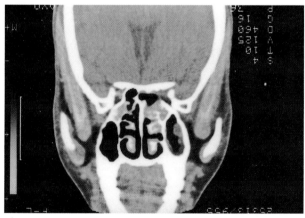

**Figure 11.24** *CT scan demonstrating successful removal of the medial orbital wall.*

operation. The anterior third of the optic canal is easily decompressed by this technique. Care should be taken to avoid damaging the ophthalmic artery. More extensive decompression is usually not necessary, but may be accomplished if the exposure is adequate. The transition from orbital apex to optic nerve is usually quite evident. The dura at the orbital apex may then be incised and the incision extended over the intracanalicular optic nerve (Fig. 11.23). Incision of the optic nerve dura is optional, probably not necessary, and the author rarely performs it.

After adequate optic nerve decompression has been accomplished, hemostasis is obtained using cottonoids soaked in oxymetazoline, and the sphenoid sinus loosely packed with oxymetazoline-soaked Vaseline gauze. The packing will be removed

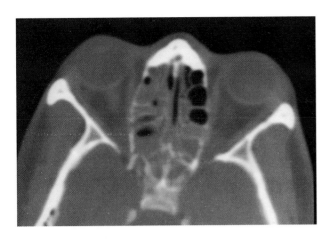

**Figure 11.25** *CT scan demonstrating a fracture of the medial wall of the optic canal.*

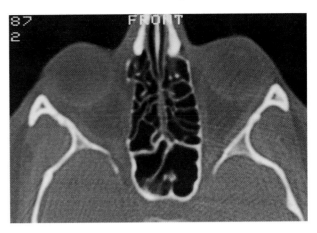

**Figure 11.26** *CT scan demonstrating a fracture of the lateral wall of the optic canal.*

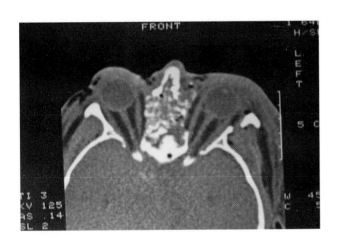

**Figure 11.27** *CT scan demonstrating extensive bony disruption of the mid-face accompanied by optic canal fractures.*

from the nose and sinus the following morning. After hemostasis has been obtained, the medial canthal tendon is reapproximated with a 5-0 Prolene suture (Ethicon, Sommerville, NJ) if it had been transected, or if it was removed with the periosteum, the periosteum is reapproximated with a 5-0 Dexon (Davis-Geck, Manatic, PR) or comparable suture. A similar suture is used to approximate the subcutaneous

tissue, and the skin is closed with 6-0 mild chromic gut. The wound is compressed with Telfa and a dental roll. Successful optic canal decompression can be documented by postoperative computed tomography (Fig. 11.24).

## COMPLICATIONS

The dreaded, potentially lethal complication of extracranial optic canal decompression is inadvertent injury to the carotid artery. This has not, to the author's knowledge been reported, but is a potential hazard. The carotid bulge may be identified inferior and lateral within the wall of the sphenoid sinus. The surgeon should stay superior while curetting and thinning the optic canal from the annulus towards the middle cranial fossa. The medial wall of the optic canal may be removed without endangering the carotid artery. The sphenoid sinus mucosa should be removed carefully, for in some sinuses the bony wall over the carotid artery is absent posteriorly.

Inadvertent entry into the anterior or middle cranial fossa may result in a CSF leak which should be repaired intraoperatively. Careful evaluation of coronal CT scans demonstrates those patients with thin ethmoid roofs. These patients are most susceptible to inadvertent entry into the anterior cranial fossa.

## COMMENT

The author's team treat all patients with traumatic optic neuropathy with a course of megadose corticosteroids as previously described. In the series of 90 patients with either pure or complex traumatic optic neuropathies, those patient with initial visual acuities of 20/100 or better had markedly improved visual function on this regimen. These patients are not candidates for extracranial optic canal decompression. ECOCD is offered to patients with visual acuity of 20/200 or worse who fail to improve after 24–48 hours of treatment with intravenous corticosteroids. Surgery is also offered to those patients who had an initial improvement in visual function while treated with the megadose corticosteroids but subsequently had deterioration in vision after the steroids were tapered or discontinued.

## OPTIC CANAL FRACTURES

Computer tomography may or may not demonstrate a variety of optic canal fractures (Figs. 11.25–11.27) in patients with traumatic optic neuropathy. In the author's experience with 60 patients with classic traumatic optic neuropathy, eight had CT evidence for optic canal fracture. All patients received a course of megadose corticosteroids. Some patients also underwent ECOCD. The presence or absence of a fracture had no predictive value as to visual outcome. There was no significant difference between visual outcome after medical or surgical treatment between patients with and without optic canal fractures.

The presence or absence of an optic canal fracture on CT does not alter the treatment plan in any way. All patients are initially treated with megadose corticosteroids with surgical options offered as discussed previously.

## SUMMARY

Trauma to the optic nerve may be obvious and untreatable or occult and treatable. It should be sought in any patient with unexplained visual dysfunction after an even trivial injury to the craniofacial region. Unexplained visual loss and a relative afferent pupillary defect indicate that the optic nerve has been traumatized. Obviously treatable etiologies, for example, an orbital hemorrhage, should be diagnosed and promptly treated. There is no consensus as to the appropriate treatment for traumatic optic neuropathies without an obviously treatable etiology. Most agree that intravenous megadose corticosteroids are a reasonable first-line treatment. There is less agreement as to the role of optic canal decompression. A randomized study is presently under way to compare the visual results of patients treated with steroids with those treated with steroids and surgery. Although steroid treatment has not been proven effective in a randomized study, the National Eye Institute thought it inappropriate to include a nontreated control group in this study.

Interestingly, recent laboratory studies have indicated that steroids may actually harm the visual outcome in rats undergoing crush injuries to their optic nerves. At this time there is no consensus as to the appropriateness of any treatment regimen for patients with traumatic optic neuropathies.[12] However, until hard data prove differently, the author's experience[17] and that of others,[15–18] indicates that patients treated with a combination of corticosteroids and optic canal decompression have a better visual prognosis than those receiving no treatment.

## REFERENCES

1 Anderson RL, Panje WR, Gross CE. Optic nerve blindness following blunt forehead trauma. *Ophthalmology* 1982; **89**: 445–55.

2 Gjerris F. Traumatic lesions of the visual pathways. In: Vinken PJ, Bruyn CW, eds. *Handbook of Clinical Neurology, Vol. 24* (Amsterdam: North Holland Publishing, 1976): 27–57.

3 Holt GR, Holt JE. Incidence of eye injuries in facial fractures: an analysis of 727 cases. *Otolaryngol Head Neck Surg* 1983; **91**: 276–9.

4 Turner JWA. Indirect injury to the optic nerves. *Brain* 1943; **66**: 140–51.

5 Corder DM, Spoor TC, Balok EM. Ocular injuries in blunt facial trauma: epidemiology and predictors of serious globe complications. *Invest Ophthalmol Vis Sci* 1991; **32(4)**: 885–6.

6 Liu D. A simplified technique of orbital decompression for

severe retrobulbar hemorrhage. *Am J Ophthalmol* 1993; **116**: 34–7.

7  Ramocki JM, Spoor TC, McHenry JG. Visual outcome in traumatic orbital hemorrhages. *Invest Ophthalmol Vis Sci* 1993; **34(4)**: 1115–16.

8  Katz B, Carmody R. Subperiosteal orbital hematoma induced by the Valsalva maneuver. *Am J Ophthalmol* 1985; **100(4)**: 617–18.

9  Hupp SL, Buckley EG, Byrne SF et al. Post-traumatic venous obstructive retinopathy associated with an enlarged optic nerve sheath. *Arch Ophthalmol* 1984; **102**: 254–6.

10 Braughler JM, Hall E. Current applications of high dose steroid therapy for CNS injury. *J Neurosurg* 1985; **62**: 806–10.

11 Bracken MB, Shepard MJ, Collins WF et al. A randomized controlled trial of methylprednisolone or naloxone in the treatment of acute spinal cord injury. *NEJM* 1990; **322**: 1405–11.

12 Bracken MD, Shepard MJ, Collins WF et al. Methylprednisolone or naloxone treatment after acute spinal cord injury: 1 year follow-up data. *J Neurosurg* 1992; **76**: 23–31.

13 Steinsapir KD, Goldberg RA. Traumatic optic neuropathy. *Surv Ophthalmol* 1994; **38**: 487–518.

14 Spoor TC, Hartel WC, Lensink DB et al. Treatment of traumatic optic neuropathy with corticosteroids. *Am J Ophthalmol* 1990; **110**: 665–9.

15 Joseph MP, Lessell S, Rizzo J, Momose J. Extracranial optic canal decompression for traumatic optic neuropathy. *Arch Ophthalmol* 1990; **108**: 1091–3.

16 Miller NR. Management of traumatic optic neuropathy. *Arch Ophthalmol* 1990; **108**: 1086–7.

17 Warner JE, Lessell S. Traumatic optic neuropathy. *Int Ophthalmol Clin* 1995; **35**: 57–62.

18 Spoor TC, McHenry JG. Management of traumatic optic neuropathy. *J Craniomaxillofac Trauma* 1996; **2**: 14–20.

# *Chapter 12* **Appendix: Ophthalmologic emergencies**

## CHEMICAL BURN (Fig. 12.1)

Immediate, copious irrigation with whatever nontoxic liquid is available.

## CENTRAL RETINAL ARTERY OCCLUSION (CRAO) (Fig. 12.2)

Occlusion of the central retinal artery may be the sequela of orbital trauma and hemorrhage (Fig. 12.3). This may be readily reversible by immediate cantho-tomy and cantholysis (Fig. 12.4). Canthotomy/cantholysis must be done aggressively, completely disinserting the lateral canthal tendons (Fig. 12.4).

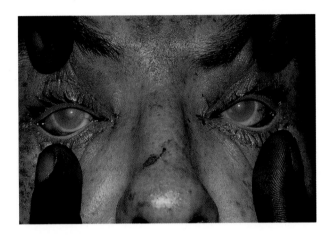

**Figure 12.1** *Alkali burn to both eyes shortly after vigorous irrigation.*

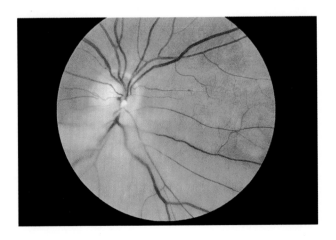

**Figure 12.2** *Central retinal artery occlusion: inferior branch of the central retinal artery is occluded by a cholesterol embolus.*

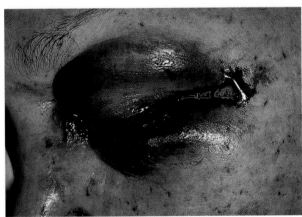

**Figure 12.3** *Severe orbital hemorrhage causing a central retinal artery occlusion.*

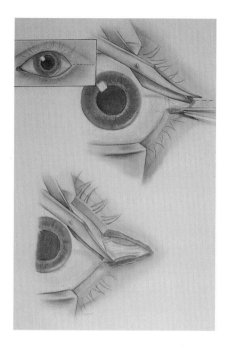

**Figure 12.4** *Canthotomy and cantholysis.*

If canthotomy/cantholysis is unsuccessful in restoring ocular circulation, the hemorrhage may be evacuated with a needle (Figs 12.5 (a)–(c)) or the orbit decompressed with a hemostat.

Classic treatment for spontaneous CRAO entails anterior chamber paracentesis, ocular massage, rebreathing air or breathing 5% carbon dioxide to dilate the retinal vessels and expel the embolus downstream. These are rarely successful, but should be tried if the patient is seen in a timely fashion.

Remember that the CRAO secondary to orbital hemorrhage is a much more treatable entity than the CRAO secondary to arterial occlusion or embolization.

## TRAUMATIC OPTIC NEUROPATHY

Patients with traumatic optic nerve injuries should be treated as soon as possible with an intravenous bolus (over 30 minutes) of 30 mg/kg methylprednisolone

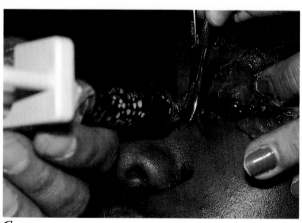

*a*

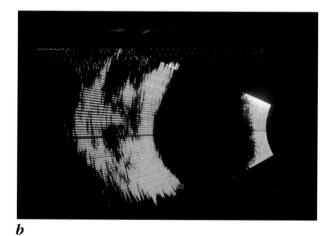

*b*

**Figure 12.5** *Orbital hemorrhage (a) localized with B-scan ultrasonography (b) (note needle opacity centered in sonolucent hemorrhage) and drained with a 22-gauge needle (c).*

*C*

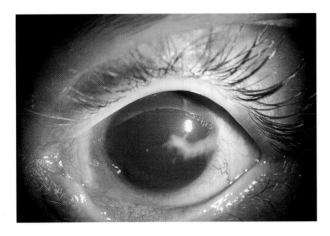

**Figure 12.6** *Traumatic hyphema.*

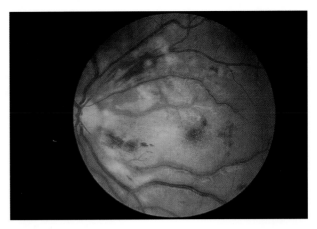

**Figure 12.7** *Disruption of posterior pole circulation after ocular trauma resulting in infarction and hemorrhage.*

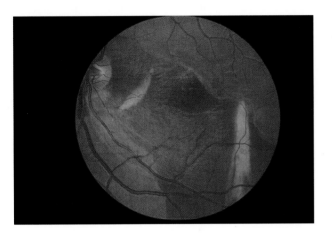

**Figure 12.8** *Choroidal tears after blunt injury to the eye.*

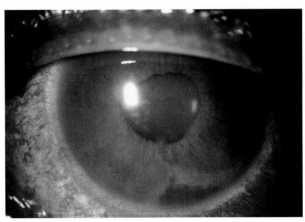

**Figure 12.9** *Microhyphema.*

(Solumedrol, Pharmacia-Upjohn, Kalamazoo MI, USA). Steroids are most effective if administered within 8 hours of injury. Two hours after the initial bolus, another bolus of 15 mg/kg methylprednisolone is given. Methylprednisolone 15 mg/kg is then administered every 6 hours for 24–48 hours. Further treatment is discussed in Chapter 11.

## TRAUMATIC HYPHEMA (Fig. 12.6)

Common errors

— failure to rule out associated injuries accounting for decreased vision (traumatic optic neuropathy, maculopathies) (Figs 12.7 and 12.8).
— failure to detect microhyphemas (Fig. 12.9), to carry out gonioscopy and to look for hemorrhage in inferior angle.

— failure to restrict activities, that is, returning the patient to a potentially dysfunctional environment.

## TREATMENT OF TRAUMATIC HYPHEMA

- Bedrest, patch
- Antifibrinolytics for high-risk patients
- Daily monitoring of intraocular pressure
- Benign neglect for uncomplicated hyphema
- Aggressive medical and surgical management for hyphema complicated by elevated intraocular pressure
- Careful indirect ophthalmoscopy 3 weeks after injury to detect and treat peripheral retinal trauma

## TRAUMATIC IRITIS

— Dilatation and cycloplegia are necessary to make sure all synechiae between the iris and the anterior lens capsule are broken.
— Topical corticosteroids by decreasing ocular inflammation may make it easier to break synechiae on a subsequent visit.
— If synechiae are not all broken after the first visit, it can be tried again after 24 hours of topical steroid treatment.

## TRAUMATIC GLAUCOMA

— Gonioscopy to detect angle recession.
— Warn patient that lifelong follow-up is necessary to detect potential post-traumatic glaucomas.
— Routinely check intraocular pressures after injury.
— Remember types of post-traumatic glaucomas—ghost cell glaucoma, angle recession glaucoma etc.

## AVOIDING MISMANAGEMENT OF OPHTHALMIC TRAUMA

The most frequent error encountered when dealing with nonophthalmologists managing periorbital injuries is failure to obtain an ophthalmologic consul-tation or failure to listen to the consultant's suggestions. It is very distressing to be asked to evaluate bilateral ruptured globes that were undetected prior to craniofacial surgery and are unsalvageable because they were not treated in a timely fashion. Such neglect of the basic eye examination is indefensible.

Failure to respond appropriately to an emergent situation—wishing it away—is a common error made by those not familiar with managing the traumatized patient. An example would be the patient with visual loss caused by optic nerve compression secondary to an orbital hemorrhage. The orbit must be decompressed until there is evidence that the optic nerve compression has been relieved, that is, lessening of the relative afferent pupillary defect. Another common error occurs when well trained, competent clinicians view the patient through their own specialty and neglect the whole picture. These errors are easily avoided if you remember that there is no substitute for a complete eye examination; and if the visual function is abnormal, a relative afferent pupillary defect (or inverse RAPD) (Fig. 12.18) should be looked for prior to dilating the patient's pupils.

## ERRORS OF OMISSION

— **Failure to document visual acuity prior to treating any ocular injury except a caustic burn**
— **Failure to examine the eye prior to periocular or orbital surgery**

A complete ophthalmologic examination is a prerequisite prior to any surgery in the periorbital region. The medical and legal importance of documenting ocular injury prior to surgery in the periorbital region is obvious.

— **Failure to differentiate visual loss due to traumatic optic neuropathy from retinal etiologies**

This can be avoided by looking carefully for a relative afferent pupillary defect or inverse afferent pupillary defect prior to dilating the pupils. After dilatation, careful examination of the retina will ascertain retinal etiologies for visual loss.

— **Macular hemorrhages**

Preretinal hemorrhages often seen after Valsalva maneuvers (weight-lifting) may cause sudden, severe loss of vision (Fig. 12.10). These will eventually

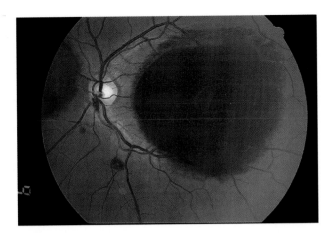

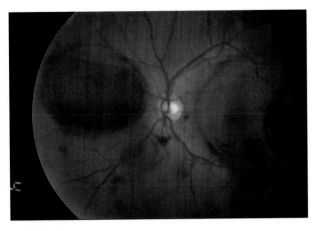

**Figure 12.10** *Subhyaloid hemorrhage after Valsalva maneuver obscuring the macula.*

**Figure 12.11** *Same patient after treatment with YAG laser. Note dispersion of hemorrhage and clearing of the macula.*

reabsorb, but vision may be restored much more quickly by treating the hemorrhage with YAG laser and dissipating it into the vitreous (Fig. 12.11).

### — Neglecting the levator when repairing a lacerated eyelid

A man received a knife wound to his upper eyelid lateral canthus and eye (Figs 12.12 (a) and (b)). After repairing the lacerated globe, the brow and eyelid wound were repaired, neglecting the lacerated levator (Fig. 12 (c)). Ptosis of the right upper eyelid was evident after surgery (Fig. 12.12 (d)). Exploration of the eyelid and advancement of the previously neglected levator obviated the ptosis (Fig. 12.12 (e)).

### — Failure to detect and repair injured canaliculi

Any injury to the medial canthal region can involve one or both canaliculi until proven otherwise. Failure to detect and repair canalicular lacerations (Figs 12.13 and 12.14) leads to chronic epiphora and necessitates conjunctival DCR with Pyrex tube placement (Fig. 12.15). Often multiple procedures are necessary. Failure to detect and repair a lacerated medial canthal tendon results in traumatic telecanthus (Fig. 12.16). These injuries may be accompanied by injury to the lacrimal sac and canaliculi.

### — Neglecting eyecare in a seriously injured patient

When caring for unconscious patients, it is important to protect their eyes. Corneal erosions secondary to drying due to incomplete eyelid closure are prone to infection by the gram-negative organisms that are ubiquitous in the intensive care unit (ICU) environment (Figs 12.17 (a)–(c)). These injuries are better prevented than treated.

### — Failure to detect (look for) traumatic injury to the optic nerve

If the degree of visual loss does not correlate with the ocular findings, a traumatic optic neuropathy should be considered. The boy in Fig. 12.18 presented with decreased vision to the level of hand motions after a BB (shotgun) injury to the left orbit. Ocular examination was normal except for a trace iritis and peripheral retinal contusion. The patient was dilated before the pupils were examined. The next day an obvious afferent pupillary defect was evident (Figs 12.18 (a) and (b)). CT scan demonstrated apical orbital compression by a BB (Fig. 12.19). Decompression of the orbital apex improved visual function.

### — Failure to detect an intraocular foreign body

The man in Fig. 12.20 was striking metal on metal while working on his tractor and noted a foreign-body sensation in his right eye. The next day he was referred with a blind, painful eye due to panophthalmitis (Fig. 12.21). The causative organism was *Bacillus cereus*.

History, history, history: what was the patient doing at the time of injury? Was there a metal-on-metal type of injury?

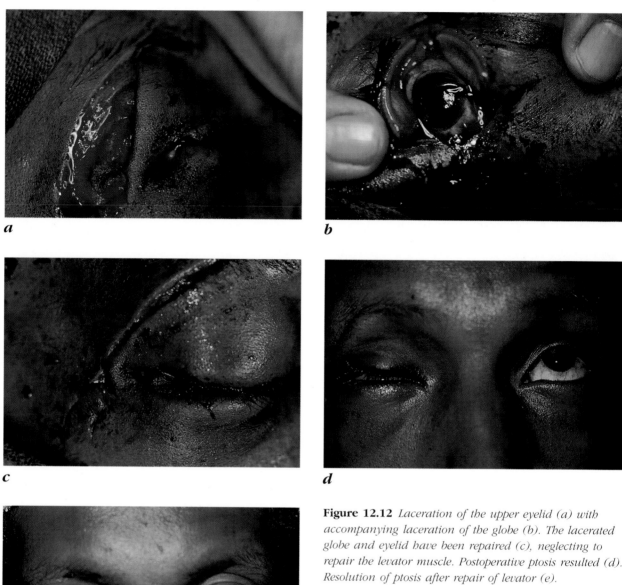

**Figure 12.12** *Laceration of the upper eyelid (a) with accompanying laceration of the globe (b). The lacerated globe and eyelid have been repaired (c), neglecting to repair the levator muscle. Postoperative ptosis resulted (d). Resolution of ptosis after repair of levator (e).*

Transilluminate iris to detect subtle penetrations.

Gonioscopy—look for foreign body in the anterior chamber angle, especially inferiorly.

Careful ophthalmoscopy by the initial examiner may detect an occult intraocular foreign body better than all the subsequent imaging studies. As in bridge, one peak is worth two finesses.

CT scans may be very helpful in detecting intraocular foreign bodies or occult ruptured globes. Only the plaintiff's attorneys will thank you for not obtain-

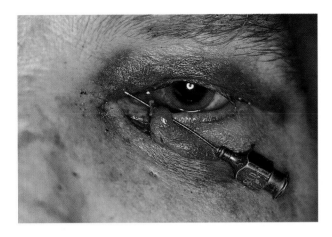

**Figure 12.13** *Laceration of the lower canaliculus.*

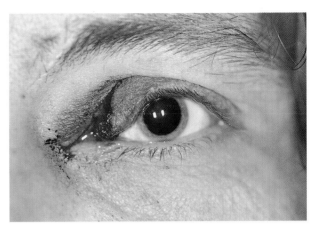

**Figure 12.14** *Laceration of the upper canaliculus.*

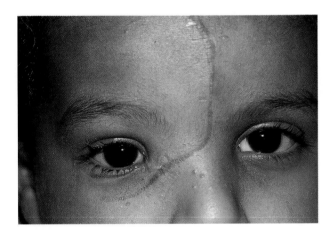

**Figure 12.15** *Patient with persistent epiphora secondary to failure to repair an occult laceration of both canaliculi after an avulsion injury.*

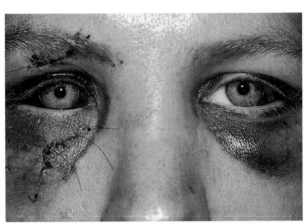

**Figure 12.16** *Traumatic telecanthus after failure to detect and repair a medical canthal tendon laceration.*

ing appropriate, or possibly appropriate, imaging studies.

## REPAIRING A RUPTURED GLOBE

An injured eye is ruptured until proven otherwise. Hints that the globe is ruptured include markedly decreased vision, deep anterior chamber, low intraocular pressure, extensive hyphema, or vitreous hemorrhage.

It is not a sin to explore a globe that is not ruptured. The small risk of general anesthesia is certainly worth the benefit of detecting and treating an occult laceration (Fig. 12.22).

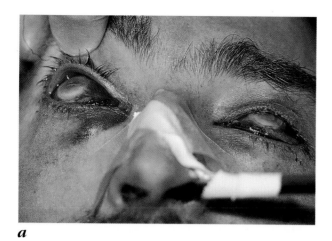

*a*

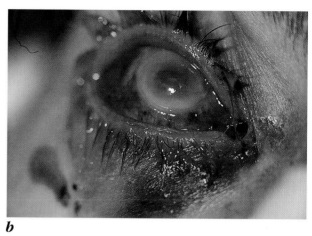

*b*

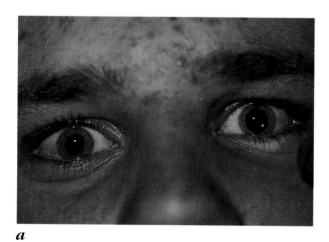

*c*

**Figure 12.17** *A patient with severe systemic injuries and neglected eye care (a), leading to corneal erosion (b) and ulceration (c). These injuries are better prevented than treated.*

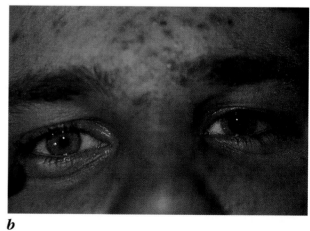

*a*

*b*

**Figure 12.18** *An inverse relative afferent pupillary defect evident in a patient with decreased vision caused by a BB injury to the left orbit (Fig. 12.19). Illumination of the affected eye causes dilatation of both pupils (a). When the normal eye is illuminated, the unaffected pupil mioses (b).*

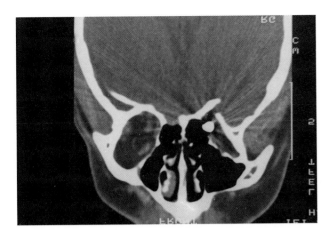

**Figure 12.19** CT scan demonstrates apical orbital compression by a BB.

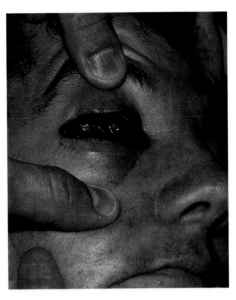

**Figure 12.20** Panophthalmitis caused by *Bacillus cereus.*

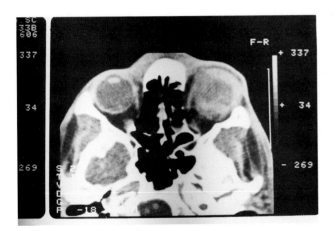

**Figure 12.21** CT scan demonstrates panophthalmitis of the right eye.

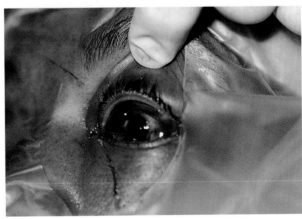

**Figure 12.22** Occult laceration of the globe caused by an apparent fingernail laceration of the eyelid.

Putting toxic drops into an open eye—preservatives, gentamycin—may significantly damage the corneal endothelium and be toxic to the retina.

Intraoperative pupillary mydriasis with intracameral instillation of intracardiac epinephrine diluted 10:1 with balanced salt solution (BSS) yields preservative-free pupillary dilatation. The pupil may be easily miosed with intracameral acetylcholine (Miochol) and Carbachol (Miostat).

Do not be afraid to replace sutures. There is nothing sacred about the sutures that you initially placed. If the sutures are poorly positioned—inappropriate depth, inappropriate length, incarcerate iris or vitreous—take them out and replace them.

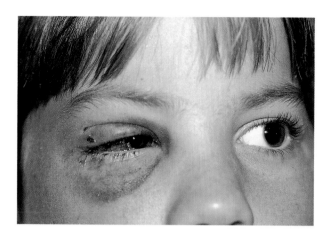

**Figure 12.23** *A boy shot with a pellet in the right orbit. Visual function was unimpaired.*

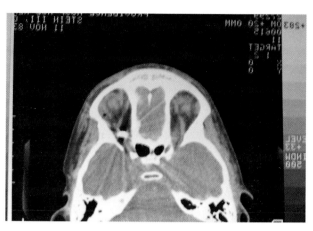

**Figure 12.24** *CT scan demonstrates pellet in the orbital apex.*

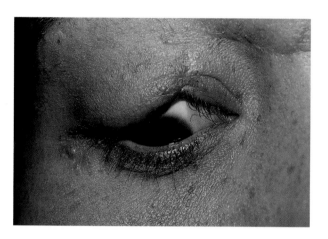

**Figure 12.25** *Notching of the upper eyelid caused by inadequate repair.*

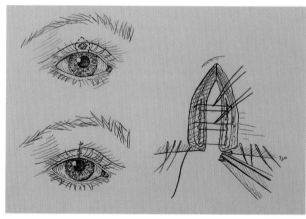

**Figure 12.26** *Proper method for excising and repairing an upper eyelid laceration utilizes three marginal and several tarsal sutures.*

Remember that nylon sutures should be placed to the level of Descemet's membrane or full thickness through the cornea.

Remember to bury the knots on the nylon sutures. Your patient will be much more comfortable postoperatively.

Prophylactic broad-spectrum intravenous antibiotic coverage is appropriate and should be used judiciously, as should topical and periocular antibiotics.

## ERRORS OF COMMISSION

The boy in Fig. 12.23 was shot in the orbit with a BB gun. There was no evidence for optic nerve compression. CT scan (Fig. 12.24) demonstrated a BB in the posterior, superior orbit. Two general ophthalmologists spent a long afternoon unsuccessfully and unnecessarily exploring the orbit.

If optic nerve function is not compromised, there is no reason to explore the orbit to remove a metallic foreign body. Even in skilled hands, it is likely that more harm will be caused than good accomplished.

## EYELID NOTCHING

Careful primary repair of an eyelid laceration will obviate late lid notching and its resultant corneal complications and the need for further surgery (Fig. 12.25). Repair the eyelid margin with three marginal sutures of 6-0 silk (Fig. 12.26).

Use two 6-0 Vicryl sutures to approximate the lower lid tarsus. Use three 6-0 Vicryl sutures to approximate the upper eyelid tarsus.

If both upper and lower eyelid lacerations are present (Fig. 12.27), consider splinting the lids with a tarsorrhaphy or with traction sutures. Remember to identify and repair the levator muscle.

Management of ocular, orbital and adnexal trauma may be challenging and rewarding. It is also fraught

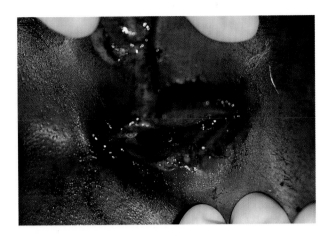

**Figure 12.27** Laceration of both upper and lower eyelids.

with potential medical and legal complications. You must remember to expect the worst until proven otherwise, examine the eye carefully, and to obtain appropriate, timely consultations.

# Index

Page numbers in italics refer to illustrations.

abscess
  corneal ring  63, *63*, *64*
  intraorbital  137, *139*
  subperiosteal orbital  *132*, 133, 137, 138, *139*
acceleration/deceleration injuries  180, *182*
accidents  20
accommodative insufficiency  107–11
acid burns  45, 46, *46*
adhesive tape allergy  *133*, 134
airbag injuries  39–40, *40*, *41*
air embolization  58
airgun injuries  123, 126–7, *128*, *129*
alkali burns  45, *45*, 46, 49–50, *49*, *191*
allergy, adhesive tape  *133*, 134
amniotic fluid embolization  58
animal bites  88–90, *88*
anterior chamber
  in chemical injuries  46
  collapse  *29*, 32
  in endophthalmitis  60, *60*
anterior cranial fossa  2, 115, 187
anterior segment injuries  35–43
antibiotics
  bite injuries  87, 90
  corneal abrasions  14, 15
  endophthalmitis prophylaxis  9–10, 22, 64
  endophthalmitis treatment  64
  gonococcal conjunctivitis  12
  medial orbital wall fractures  12
  orbital cellulitis  138–40
antifibrinolytic agents  41
aqueous fluid, specimen collection  62
assaults, chemicals  *49*, 50

*Bacillus cereus* endophthalmitis  *9*, 10, 62–4, *62–4*, 195,
    *199*
ballistics  120–7
BB pellet injuries  54, 126, 200, *200*
bed rest  42
birdshot  *30*, 126
bites
  animal  88–90, *88*
  human  87, *88*
  insect  *133*, 134

blunt trauma
  anterior segment  35–43
  orbital fractures  153, *153*
  posterior segment  51–7
  ruptured globe  *21*, 28–32, 35, *36*
bullet wounds  120–7, *127*
burns *see* chemical injuries; thermal injuries

canaliculi
  injuries  77, *77*, *78*, 195, *197*
  repair  78–80, *79*
canthotomy/cantholysis
  central retinal artery occlusion  191, *192*
  lower eyelid repair  70–2, *72*
  orbital floor fractures  *160*, 161
  orbital hemorrhage  147, 169, 178–9, *178–9*
  upper eyelid repair  85, *87*
  *see also* lateral canthotomy
carotid artery, inadvertant injury  187
carotid-cavernous fistula  11, *18*, 20, 142–3, *144–5*
  cranial nerve palsies  107, *110*
cataract  37, *38*, 46
cavernous sinus  2, *101*
  thrombosis  137, *140*
cellulitis, orbital *see* orbital cellulitis
central retinal artery occlusion  177–8, *178*, 191–2, *191*
chemical injuries  45–50
  effects  46
  grading of severity  47–8, *47*
  immediate management  4, 45–6, 191
  prognosis  48–50
  surgical management  46–7
chemosis, subconjunctival hemorrhagic  7, *7*, 12, *12*,
    29–30, *29*
child abuse  60, *60*, 149, *151*
childbirth  58, 60
children
  orbital cellulitis  138–40
  transient cortical blindness  101
chorioretinal rupture  54
choroid
  neovascularization  53–4, *53*
  rupture  52–4, *52–3*
  tears  38–9, *38*, *193*

commotio retinae 39, *39*, 51–2, *51*, *52*
compression injuries 58
computed tomography (CT) scan
    intraocular foreign body 16, *16*
    orbital fractures 154–5, 156–8
    orbital inflammation 132–5
    penetrating orbital injuries 117, *117*, 128
    ruptured globe 7, *7*, *29–30*, 32
concomitant deviations 107, *111*
conjunctiva
    recession surgery 46
    transplantation 46
conjunctivitis 11–12
    acute purulent gonococcal 11–12, *11*
connective tissue diseases 58
contrecoup injury 51
convergence insufficiency 107–11, *111*
cornea
    abrasion 12–15, *13–15*
    blood-staining 42, *43*
    blunt trauma 35–6
    burn injuries *45*, 46, *46*
    decompensation 37–8, *37*
    erosions 195, *198*
    foreign body 12–15, *13–14*
    grafting 48, *48*
    laceration 26, *26*
        complex 26–7, *27*, *28*
        repair 26, *27*
    ring abscess 63, *63*, 64
    ulcers, infected 12, *13*
corneal-scleral laceration 25–6, *25–6*
corneoscleral rupture 35, *36*
corticosteroids
    optic neuropathy 170–2, 179, 180–3, 188, 192–3
    orbital floor fractures 156, 157
    orbital inflammation 132, 142
    penetrating orbital injuries 118, 119
coup injury 51
cranial nerves *101*, 103
    isolated palsies 103–7
    multiple palsies 107, *109*
    penetrating injuries 120, *121*
Crawford canalicular intubation system 78–80, *79*
CSF leaks 185–6, 187
CT scan *see* computed tomography (CT) scan
cyanoacrylate glue 27
cyclodialysis 36–7

dacryoadenitis 141, *142*
dacryocystitis 77, *77*
dacryocystorhinostomy (DCR) 77, *77*, 78, 80
    conjunctival (cDCR) 77, *77*, 78
Descemet's membrane, tears 36
diabetes mellitus 140
diplopia
    cranial nerve palsies 103–4, 105–6
    medial orbital wall fractures *166*, 167

orbital floor fractures 155, 156–8
    residual, after orbital fracture repair 172–3, *172*
dysthyroid orbitopathy 141–2, *143*

ecchymosis, periorbital 159, *159*
ectropion 90–1
    lower eyelid 70, *71*, 74
    treatment 91, *91*
    upper eyelid 90, *90*
emergencies, ophthalmologic 191–201
emphysema, orbital *3*, 12, *13*, 153, *153*, 167
endophthalmitis 17–18, 60–4
    antibiotic prophylaxis 9–10, 22, 64
    endogenous 60–1, *61*
    exogenous 60
    intraocular foreign body and 8, *9*, 16–17, *16–17*, 18,
        63–4, *63–4*
    postoperative 61–2, *61*
    signs and symptoms 11, 60
    traumatic 62–4
    treatment 64
enophthalmos *154*, 155, 157, *157*, 167
enucleation 3–4, 32
epiphora 77, *77*
epsilon-amino caproic acid (Amicar) 41
errors, management
    avoiding 194
    of commission 200–1
    of omission 194–7
ethmoidectomy, external 184–5, *184*
ethmoid sinus 1, 2, 115
ethmoid sinusitis 136, *136*
examination, initial 4–8, 194
exotropia 111, *111*
extracranial transethmoidal optic canal decompression
    (ECOCD) 183–7, *184–6*, 188
    complications 187
extraocular muscles
    dysfunction 103–7
    entrapment 156–7, 159–60, *159*, 173
    *see also individual muscles*
eyecare, neglected 195, *198*
eye examination, initial 4–8, 194
eyelids
    bite injuries 87–90, *88*
    injuries 67–94
        with ruptured globe 27, *28*
        secondary repair 91–4
    notching 68, *68*, *69*, 92, 201
    in orbital cellulitis 136
    suturing together 169
    thermal injuries 48, 49, 67, *68*, 88–9, 90–1
    *see also* lateral canthus; lower eyelid; medial canthus;
        upper eyelid
eyewear, protective 20, 50

fluorescein stain 13, *14*
foreign body

corneal 12–15, *13–14*
  intraocular *see* intraocular foreign body
  orbital 117–18, *118*, 120, 126–7, 200–1
fourth cranial nerve *101*, 103
  palsy *102*, 103–5
fractures
  long bone 58
  orbit 153–73
frozen globe 107, *110*

Gargoyle glasses 20
glaucoma
  angle-closure 11, *17*, 19
  in chemical injuries 46
  ghost cell 38, *38*
  post-traumatic 36, 194
globe
  frozen 107, *110*
  inferior displacement 159
  ruptured *see* ruptured globe
glue, cyanoacrylate 27
gonococcal conjunctivitis, acute purulent 11–12, *11*
gull-wing incision 167–8, *168*, 184, *184*
gunshot wounds *31*, 32, *116*, 120–7, *126–7*

*Haemophilus influenzae* infections 138–40
halving technique 25, *26*, 27
handguns 123
head trauma
  neuro-ophthalmologic examination 95–6
  neuro-ophthalmologic manifestations 95–113
  optic neuropathy 176
  Purtscher's retinopathy 58
hemorrhage
  intracranial 58
  macular 39, *39*, 194–5
  optic nerve sheath 148–9, *150*, 179, *182*
  orbital *see* orbital hemorrhage
  subconjunctival 12, *12*, 29–30, *29*
  vitreous *see* vitreous hemorrhage
home, burn injuries at 50
Hughes tarsoconjunctival flap procedure 73–4, *73*
human bites 87, *88*
Hummelsheim transposition procedure 106, *106*
hydrostatic pressure syndrome 58
hypertropia, left (LHT) *102*
hyphema, traumatic 36, *36*, 40–3, *42*, 193–4, *193*
  scleral rupture and 29–30
  secondary 42, *43*
  surgical management 42–3
  total (eight-ball) 42, *42*
  treatment 40–2, 194
hypopyon 60, *60*

imaging studies
  orbital inflammation 132–5
  ruptured globe 32

*see also* computed tomography (CT) scan; magnetic resonance imaging
implants, orbital 165–6, *165*, 168–9
  complications 169, 170, *171*, 172
industrial injuries 50
infections, orbital 135–40
inferior oblique, recession/myotomy *103*, 104–5
inferior rectus
  entrapment *155*, *156*, 173
  recession 105
  transposition 106, *106*
inflamed orbit *see* orbital inflammation
infraorbital nerve injuries 155–6, 160, 164
infraorbital neurovascular bundle *162*, 163–4, *164*
insect bites *133*, 134
intracranial hemorrhage 58
intracranial injuries 2, *2*, 120, *124*
intracranial pressure, elevated 105, 177–8
intraocular foreign body 15–17, *16–17*
  endophthalmitis and 8, *9*, 16–17, *16–17*, 18, 63–4, *63–4*
  failure to detect 195–7, *199*
  initial evaluation 8, *8*
intraocular pressure, in traumatic hyphema 42–3
intraorbital abscess 137, *139*
iridodialysis 36
iridodonesis *36*, 37
iritis
  intraocular foreign body causing 15–16, *15*
  traumatic 11, 18, 194
irrigation, eye 45–6, 191

keratoconjunctivitis, acute purulent gonococcal 11–12, *11*
keratopathy, suture 82, *82*
keratoprosthesis 49–50, *49*

lacrimal gland injuries 81, 82–4, *84*
lacrimal sac injuries 77, *77*
lacrimal trauma 67–94
lateral canthal tendon repair 75–6
lateral canthotomy
  repair 25, *25*
  in ruptured globe 22
  *see also* canthotomy/cantholysis
lateral canthus
  injuries 67, *69*, 74–6
  repair 74–6, *75*
  tarsal strip procedure 75–6, *75*, *76*
lateral rectus resection 106
lens
  dislocation 37–9
  removal 27
  subluxation *36*, 37–9, *37*
leukemia 149, *150*
levator muscle
  failure to repair 195, *196*
  injuries 81, *81*, 82, *83*

light-near dissociation 96
lipid peroxidation 180
lower eyelid 67
   complications of repair *71*, 74
   notching 74, 92
   primary repair 70–4, *70–2*, 201
   retraction/adhesion to orbital rim 92–4, *92*, 173, *173*
lymphangioma 149, *151*

macular hemorrhage 39, *39*, 194–5
macular hole, traumatic 54–5, *55*
magnetic resonance imaging (MRI) 96–7, 99, *100*, 127
maxillary sinus 2, 115
   in orbital fracture repair 164–5, 170
medial canthal tendon
   injuries 76–7, *77*, *168*, 173, 195, *197*
   repair 169
medial canthus *76*
   injuries 67, 76–81
   repair 80–1, *80*
   webbing *93*, 94
medial orbital wall fractures *see* orbital wall fractures, medial
medial rectus
   entrapment *166–7*, 167–9
   Oculinum treatment 106–7
   recession 106
Medpore implants 165–6, 169
mesh implants, orbit 165–6, *165*, 169
microhyphema 193, *193*
middle cranial fossa 2, 115, 187
myocutaneous flaps 85, 87
myositis, orbital *131*, 132, 134–5, *134*, 141–2, *142*

nasolacrimal duct injuries 77, *77*
near reflex, spasm of 111–12, *112*
neuro-ophthalmologic manifestations 95–113

occipital cortex trauma 97–103
Oculinum 106–7
oculomotor nerves *101*, 103
   penetrating injuries 120, *121*
   *see also* fourth cranial nerve; sixth cranial nerve
ophthalmia, sympathetic 32
ophthalmoplegia 118–19, *119*, *120*
OPS needle 25, *25*
optic atrophy 176, *176*
   sector 95–6, *96*
optic canal 2
   extracranial transethmoidal decompression (ECOCD) 183–7, *184–6*, 188
   fractures *187*, 188
   skeletal deformation 180, *183*
optic chiasm 2
   injuries 96–7
optic disc, in optic neuropathy 176, *176*
optic nerve
   mechanisms of injury 179–80

transection/avulsion 175, *175–6*
optic nerve sheath
   decompression 148–9, 179, *182*
   hemorrhage 148–9, *150*, 179, *182*
optic neuropathy, traumatic 39, 96, *97*, 175–85
   after orbital surgery 169–72
   avoiding mismanagement 194
   complex 175
   corticosteroid therapy 170–2, 179, 180–3, 188, 192–3
   failure to diagnose 195, *198–9*
   incidence 176
   initial examination 5–6
   management 177–88, 192–3
   in orbital emphysema 167
   in orbital hemorrhage 177–8, *178*
orbit
   anatomic relations 1–2, *1*
   complications of surgery 169–73
   foreign body 117–18, *118*, 120, 126–7, 200–1
   fractures 153–73
   infections 135–40
   penetrating injuries 115–30
   roof fractures 159
orbital apex syndrome 117–18, *123*
orbital cellulitis 134
   postseptal (true) 136–8, *138–9*
   preseptal 135–6, *135*, *136–7*, 138
   treatment 138–40
orbital floor
   decompression 147–8, 179
   fractures 35, 153–8
      indications for repair 156–8
      patient evaluation 158–60
      preseptal orbital hemorrhage 145, *146*
      repair 160–6, *160–3*, *164*, *165*
orbital hemorrhage 145–9
   central retinal artery occlusion 191–2, *191*
   management 147–9, 178–9, *178–80*, 191–2, *192*
   optic neuropathy in 177–8, *178*
   other causes 149, *150–1*
   postoperative 169
   postseptal 147–9, *148–9*
   preseptal 145, *145–6*
   subperiosteal 145–6, *147*, 179, *181*
orbital inflammation 11, *18*, 19, 131–49
   anterior 142
   idiopathic (pseudotumor) 141–2
   posterior 142, *143*
orbital rim
   eyelid adhesion to 92–4, *92*, 173, *173*
   fractures 163, *163*, *165*
orbital wall fractures, medial *3*, 12, 35, 166–9, *166–7*
   orbital emphysema in *13*, 153, *153*, 167
   repair technique 167–9, *168*
oxymetazoline (Afrin) 163, 167, 184, 186

pancreatitis, acute 58
paranasal sinuses 2, 115, *115*, *116*

paranasal sinusitis 136, *136*
parietal lobe injuries 101–3
patching, eye 14–15, *15*
pellet wounds *31*, 32, 116, *116*, 120–7, *128*, 129–30, *129*
penetrating trauma
    double 32
    orbit 115–30
    ruptured globe 21–7
perfluorocarbon liquids 57
perineuritis 141, *141*
periocular regions 67, *69*
periosteal-temporalis fascia flaps *92, 94*, 173
periscleritis *18*, 141, *141*
peritomy 22, *23*
phthisis bulbi 46
posterior segment 51–64
    nonpenetrating trauma 51–7
    in systemic trauma 57–60
proptosis 134, 137, 159
prostate carcinoma, metastatic 149, *150*
pseudo-cherry-red spot 51, *52*
pseudomyopia 111–12
ptosis
    in eyelid injuries 81, *81*, 195, *196*
    in orbital injuries 118, 119
pupillary dilatation
    in orbital surgery 169
    postoperative 170
    in ruptured globe 199
pupils
    dysfunction 96
    irregular 36
    light-near dissociation 96
    *see also* relative afferent pupillary defect
Purtscher's retinopathy 58, *58*

raccoon eyes 159, *159*
recti muscles
    scleral rupture under insertion 23–4, *24*, 32, 35, *36*
    *see also* inferior rectus; medial rectus
red eye 11
red orbit *see* orbital inflammation
relative afferent pupillary defect (RAPD) 5–6, *5*, 175–6,
    *177*, 194
    chiasmal lesions 96
    failure to detect 195, *198–9*
    inverse *5*, 6, *177*
retinal artery occlusion, central 177–8, *178*, 191–2, *191*
retinal detachment, traumatic 55–6, *56*
retinal dialysis 56, *57*
retinal hemorrhages, in infants 60
retinal tears 57
    giant 57, *57*
rifles 123
ruptured globe 3, *4*, 21–32, 126–7
    associated injuries 27, *28*
    in blunt trauma *21*, 28–32, 35, *36*
    exploration for suspected 32

imaging studies 32
initial examination 6, 7
occult 12, *12*, 31–2
operative repair 22–7, 197–200
prognosis 8–9, *10*, 21
prophylactic antibiotics 9–10, 22
sympathetic ophthalmia 32
timing of surgery 10–11, 21–2

safety glasses 20
sclera
    lacerations 22–5, *23–4*
    occult rupture 30–1, 32
sclopetaria 54, *54*
self-destructive personalities *19*, 20
seventh cranial nerve palsy *102*, 105–6
shaken baby syndrome 60, *60*
shotgun injuries 54, *117*, 123–6, *125*
sickle cell trait 41
sinusitis, paranasal 136, *136*
sixth cranial nerve *101*, 103
    palsy *102, 104*, 105–7, *105–6, 111*
skin grafts
    ectropion repair 90, *91*
    eyelid injuries 70, 85, *85*
sliding tarsoconjunctival flap 73–4, *73*
sliding Tenzel flap 72–3, *72*
sodium hydroxide assaults *49*, 50
spasm of near reflex 111–12, *112*
specimen collection, in endophthalmitis 62
sports injuries 20
*Staphylococcus* endophthalmitis 10
*Staphylococcus epidermidis* 61, *61*, 62
steroids *see* corticosteroids
subconjunctival hemorrhage 12, *12*, 29–30, *29*
subperiosteal orbital abscess *132*, 133, 137, 138, *139*
subperiosteal orbital hemorrhage 145–6, *147*, 179, *181*
succinyl choline 22
superior oblique palsy *102*, 103–5
superior rectus transposition 106, *106*
suture keratopathy 82, *82*
sympathetic ophthalmia 32

tarsal strip procedure 75–6, *75, 76*
tarsoconjunctival flap, sliding 73–4, *73*
tattoos *19*, 20
telecanthus, traumatic 76, 77, *168*, 169, 173, 195, *197*
temporalis fascia-periosteal flaps *92, 94*, 173
temporal lobe 2
    injuries 101–3
tenonplasty 46–7
Tenzel flap 72–3, *72*
Terson's syndrome 58–9, *59*
thermal injuries 45–50
    eyelids *48*, 49, 67, *68*, 88–9, 90–1
    grading of severity 47–8, *47*
    prognosis 48–50
third-nerve palsy 107, *108–9, 121*

three-step test  *102*, 104
tranexamic acid  41
trimalar fractures  158–9, *162*, 163

unconscious patients, eyecare  195, *198*
upper eyelid  67, 81–5
    foreign body under  13–14, *14*
    horizontal lacerations  82–5, *83–6*
    large lacerations  85, *87–8*
    notching  82, *83*, 92, *200*, 201
    retraction and scarring  *93*, 94
    total loss  85, *87–8*
    vertical lacerations  81–2, *82*, *200*, 201
    *see also* levator muscle
uveal prolapse  22, *23*, 25–6, 32

Valsalva retinopathy  59, *59*, 194–5, *195*
visual acuity, documentation  4–5, 194
visual field defects  95–6, *95*
    occipital cortex injuries  98–9, *98*, *99*, *100*
    temporal/parietal injuries  101–3
vitrectomy
    in endophthalmitis  64
    in Terson's syndrome  58–9
vitreous
    base avulsion  56, *56*
    specimen collection  62
vitreous hemorrhage  29
    secondary to hyphema  38, *38*
    in Terson's syndrome  58–9
Vossius, ring of  38